Autoimmune Protocol Lifestyle Diet 2024

A Personalized Path to Navigating Autoimmune Conditions Through Dieting for Optimal Health and Wellness

Grace Mitchell

Table of Content

Introduction

Understanding the Autoimmune Protocol (AIP)

The Autoimmune Protocol (AIP) is a dietary approach designed to help individuals manage autoimmune conditions by reducing inflammation and supporting overall health. It's a more stringent version of the paleo diet, focusing on eliminating foods that are known to trigger inflammation and immune reactions while emphasizing nutrient-dense, healing foods.

Origins of the Autoimmune Protocol:

The AIP originated from the work of Dr. Loren Cordain, who developed the paleo diet, and further refined by Dr. Sarah Ballantyne, a medical biophysicist, and author of "The Paleo Approach." Dr. Ballantyne's extensive research into autoimmune diseases and the gut microbiome led to the development of the AIP as a therapeutic diet for managing autoimmune conditions.

Principles of the Autoimmune Protocol:

1. **Elimination of Trigger Foods:** The primary focus of the AIP is to remove foods that can trigger inflammation and immune responses in susceptible individuals. These include grains, legumes, dairy, refined sugars, processed oils, nightshade vegetables, eggs, nuts, seeds, and certain spices.

2. **Emphasis on Nutrient-Dense Foods:** The AIP encourages the consumption of nutrient-dense foods to support healing and overall health. This includes a variety of vegetables, fruits, quality meats, organ meats, wild-caught fish, bone broth, healthy fats like coconut oil and olive oil, and fermented foods.

3. **Gut Health:** The AIP places a strong emphasis on gut health, recognizing the significant role the gut plays in autoimmune conditions. It promotes the consumption of foods that support a healthy gut microbiome, such as probiotic-rich foods like fermented vegetables and bone broth.

4. **Potential for Reintroduction:** While the AIP initially involves strict elimination, it's designed to be a temporary phase. Once symptoms improve, individuals can gradually reintroduce eliminated foods to identify any triggers and create a personalized long-term approach to diet.

Conditions Managed by the Autoimmune Protocol:

The AIP is commonly used to manage various autoimmune conditions, including but not limited to:

- Rheumatoid arthritis
- Hashimoto's thyroiditis
- Lupus
- Celiac disease
- Inflammatory bowel disease (IBD)
- Psoriasis
- Multiple sclerosis
- Type 1 diabetes

Challenges and Considerations:

While the AIP can be highly beneficial for many individuals with autoimmune conditions, it can also present challenges. The strict elimination of certain foods may require careful meal planning and adjustment, especially when dining out or socializing.

Additionally, the AIP may not be suitable for everyone, and it's essential to work with a healthcare provider or nutritionist when embarking on this dietary approach, especially for those with complex medical conditions or nutritional deficiencies.

Benefits of the Autoimmune Protocol (AIP) Lifestyle Diet

The Autoimmune Protocol (AIP) Lifestyle Diet offers a comprehensive approach to managing autoimmune conditions by addressing underlying inflammation, supporting gut health, and promoting overall well-being. Here are some extensive insights into the benefits of adopting the AIP Lifestyle Diet:

1. Reduced Inflammation:

- One of the primary goals of the AIP Lifestyle Diet is to reduce inflammation in the body. By eliminating foods that commonly trigger inflammation, such as grains, dairy, and processed sugars, individuals may experience a significant reduction in inflammatory markers.
- Chronic inflammation is linked to the development and exacerbation of autoimmune conditions. By adopting an anti-inflammatory diet like AIP, individuals may experience relief from symptoms such as joint pain, fatigue, and digestive issues.

2. Improved Gut Health:

- The AIP Lifestyle Diet emphasizes foods that support a healthy gut microbiome, such as fermented foods, bone broth, and fiber-rich vegetables.
- Gut health plays a crucial role in autoimmune conditions, as imbalances in the gut microbiota can contribute to immune dysregulation and inflammation. By supporting gut health, individuals may experience improvements in their autoimmune symptoms and overall well-being.

3. Identification of Trigger Foods:

- The AIP Lifestyle Diet involves an elimination phase followed by a systematic reintroduction of foods to identify potential triggers.
- By gradually reintroducing eliminated foods, individuals can identify specific foods that exacerbate their autoimmune symptoms. This personalized approach allows for the creation of a tailored dietary plan that meets individual needs and preferences.

4. Nutrient-Dense Foods:

- The AIP Lifestyle Diet encourages the consumption of nutrient-dense foods that provide essential vitamins, minerals, and antioxidants.
- By focusing on foods such as vegetables, fruits, quality meats, and healthy fats, individuals can ensure they are meeting their nutritional needs while supporting their body's healing processes.

5. Enhanced Energy and Vitality:

- Many individuals report increased energy levels and improved vitality after adopting the AIP Lifestyle Diet.
- By eliminating foods that may cause energy crashes and fatigue, individuals can experience more sustained energy throughout the day. Additionally, the nutrient-dense nature of the diet provides the body with the fuel it needs to thrive.

6. Weight Management:

- The AIP Lifestyle Diet may support weight management goals by promoting the consumption of whole, unprocessed foods and reducing reliance on calorie-dense, nutrient-poor foods.
- Additionally, some individuals may experience reductions in bloating and water retention, leading to a slimmer, more comfortable physique.

7. Psychological Well-being:

- Improvements in physical health often translate to benefits for psychological well-being.
- By experiencing relief from symptoms and feeling more in control of their health, individuals may experience reduced stress and anxiety levels, improved mood, and enhanced overall quality of life.

Understanding How the Autoimmune Protocol (AIP) Diet Works

The Autoimmune Protocol (AIP) Diet is a therapeutic approach designed to address autoimmune diseases by focusing on reducing inflammation, healing the gut, and identifying and eliminating potential trigger foods. Here's an extensive overview of how the AIP Diet works:

1. Identification and Elimination of Trigger Foods:

- The AIP Diet begins with a strict elimination phase, during which individuals remove foods that are known to trigger inflammation and immune reactions.

- Common trigger foods eliminated during this phase include grains, legumes, dairy, processed sugars, processed oils, nightshade vegetables, eggs, nuts, seeds, and certain spices.
- By removing these potentially problematic foods from the diet, individuals aim to reduce inflammation and give their bodies a chance to heal.

2. Focus on Nutrient-Dense Foods:
- While eliminating trigger foods, the AIP Diet emphasizes the consumption of nutrient-dense, healing foods.
- This includes a wide variety of vegetables, fruits, quality meats, organ meats, wild-caught fish, bone broth, healthy fats like coconut oil and olive oil, and fermented foods.
- These nutrient-dense foods provide essential vitamins, minerals, antioxidants, and other compounds that support the body's healing processes and overall well-being.

3. Support for Gut Health:
- The AIP Diet places a strong emphasis on gut health, recognizing the significant role the gut plays in autoimmune conditions.
- Gut health is supported through the consumption of foods that promote a healthy gut microbiome, such as probiotic-rich fermented foods like sauerkraut, kimchi, and kombucha, as well as bone broth and fiber-rich vegetables.
- By promoting gut health, individuals can improve digestion, enhance nutrient absorption, and reduce intestinal permeability, which may help alleviate autoimmune symptoms.

4. Gradual Reintroduction of Foods:
- After a period of strict elimination, individuals can gradually reintroduce eliminated foods one at a time to identify any triggers.
- The reintroduction phase is done systematically, with careful observation of any changes in symptoms or overall well-being.
- By reintroducing foods methodically, individuals can identify specific triggers and create a personalized long-term approach to diet that minimizes autoimmune symptoms while maximizing dietary variety and enjoyment.

5. Lifestyle Factors:

- In addition to dietary changes, the AIP Diet often incorporates lifestyle factors that support overall health and well-being.
- This may include stress management techniques such as meditation, yoga, or deep breathing exercises, adequate sleep, regular physical activity, and minimizing exposure to environmental toxins.
- These lifestyle factors play a complementary role in supporting the body's ability to manage autoimmune conditions and promote optimal health.

6. Individualized Approach:

- It's essential to recognize that the AIP Diet is not a one-size-fits-all approach. Every individual's experience with autoimmune disease is unique, and dietary needs may vary accordingly.
- The AIP Diet encourages individuals to listen to their bodies, pay attention to how different foods affect them, and adjust their diet accordingly.
- Working with a healthcare provider or nutritionist who is knowledgeable about autoimmune conditions can help individuals navigate the AIP Diet and tailor it to their specific needs and preferences.

Foods to Avoid and Foods to Include on the Autoimmune Protocol (AIP) Diet

The Autoimmune Protocol (AIP) Diet involves eliminating certain foods that may trigger inflammation and immune reactions while emphasizing nutrient-dense, healing foods. Here's an extensive breakdown of foods to avoid and foods to include on the AIP Diet:

Foods to Avoid:

1. **Grains:** Wheat, barley, rye, oats, corn, rice, and other gluten-containing grains should be avoided due to their potential to trigger inflammation and immune reactions.
2. **Legumes:** Beans, lentils, chickpeas, peanuts, and soybeans contain compounds such as lectins and phytates that may contribute to gut inflammation and irritation.

3. **Dairy:** All forms of dairy, including milk, cheese, yogurt, and butter, should be eliminated due to their lactose and casein content, which can be problematic for individuals with autoimmune conditions.

4. **Processed Sugars:** Refined sugars, high-fructose corn syrup, and artificial sweeteners should be avoided due to their potential to disrupt blood sugar levels and contribute to inflammation.

5. **Processed Oils:** Vegetable oils such as soybean oil, corn oil, canola oil, and sunflower oil are high in omega-6 fatty acids and may promote inflammation when consumed in excess.

6. **Nightshade Vegetables:** Tomatoes, potatoes, peppers, eggplants, and spices derived from nightshade plants (such as paprika and chili powder) contain compounds known as alkaloids, which may exacerbate inflammation in some individuals.

7. **Eggs:** Eggs are a common allergen and may trigger immune reactions in susceptible individuals. They are often eliminated during the initial phase of the AIP Diet and reintroduced later to assess tolerance.

8. **Nuts and Seeds:** Nuts and seeds contain compounds such as lectins, phytates, and enzyme inhibitors that may contribute to gut irritation and inflammation. They are typically eliminated during the elimination phase of the AIP Diet and reintroduced cautiously.

9. **Spices:** Certain spices, such as cayenne pepper, chili powder, and curry powder, may contain nightshade ingredients or other compounds that can trigger inflammation and should be avoided during the elimination phase.

Foods to Include:

1. **Vegetables:** A wide variety of non-nightshade vegetables should form the foundation of the AIP Diet. This includes leafy greens, cruciferous vegetables (such as broccoli, cabbage, and Brussels sprouts), root vegetables (such as sweet potatoes, carrots, and beets), and squash.

2. **Fruits:** Berries, apples, pears, citrus fruits, and other low-glycemic fruits can provide natural sweetness and important vitamins and minerals without spiking blood sugar levels.

3. **Quality Meats:** Grass-fed beef, pasture-raised poultry, wild-caught fish, and organ meats are excellent sources of protein, iron, and other essential nutrients. Whenever feasible, use hormone-free and organic products.

4. **Healthy Fats:** Coconut oil, olive oil, avocado oil, and animal fats from pastured animals are all healthy sources of fats that can be included in moderation on the AIP Diet.

5. **Bone Broth:** Bone broth is rich in collagen, gelatin, and other healing compounds that support gut health and reduce inflammation. It can be consumed as a warm beverage or used as a base for soups and stews.

6. **Fermented Foods:** Probiotic-rich foods such as sauerkraut, kimchi, coconut yogurt, and kombucha can help support a healthy gut microbiome and improve digestion.

7. **Herbs and Spices:** While certain spices are eliminated during the elimination phase of the AIP Diet, many herbs and spices are allowed and can add flavor and variety to AIP-friendly meals. Examples include basil, oregano, thyme, rosemary, and ginger.

8. **Non-Dairy Alternatives:** Coconut milk, coconut cream, and almond milk (if tolerated) can be used as alternatives to dairy milk in AIP-friendly recipes.

1

Breakfast recipes

Turmeric Ginger Smoothie

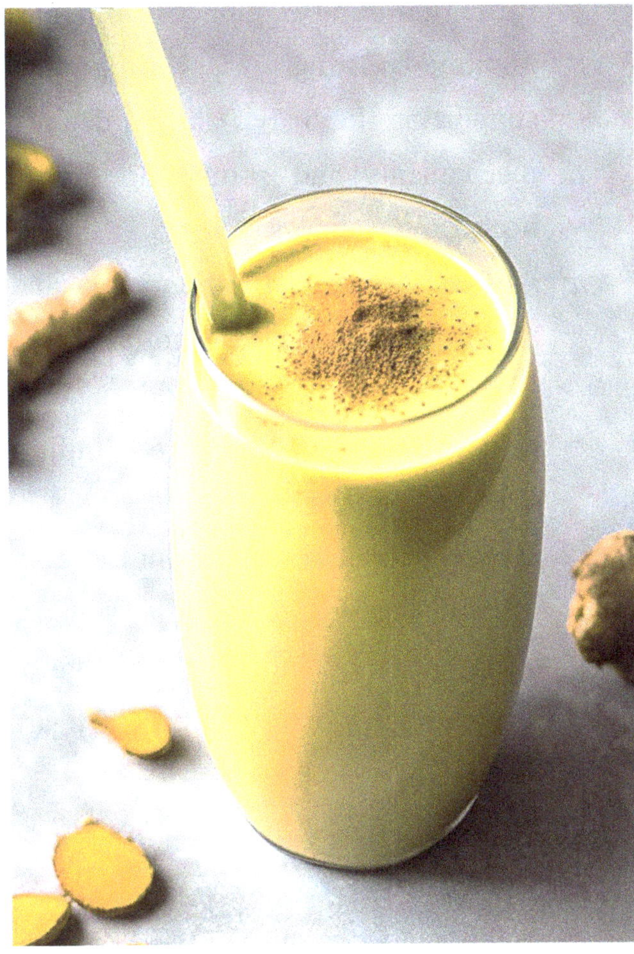

Time of Preparation: 5 minutes

Serving Units: 1

Ingredients:

- 1 ripe banana, frozen
- 1/2 cup frozen pineapple chunks
- 1/2 cup coconut milk (or any dairy-free milk of choice)
- 1/2 teaspoon ground turmeric
- 1/2 teaspoon grated fresh ginger
- One tablespoon (optional, for sweetness) of honey or maple syrup
- If desired, add 1/2 teaspoon of ground cinnamon for taste
- 1/2 cup ice cubes

Procedures:

1. After peeling, cut the banana into large pieces.
2. Grate the fresh ginger.
3. In a blender, combine the frozen banana chunks, frozen pineapple chunks, coconut milk, ground turmeric, grated ginger, honey or maple syrup (if using), ground cinnamon (if using), and ice cubes.
4. Blend on high speed until smooth and creamy, adding more coconut milk if needed to reach your desired consistency.
5. Pour the smoothie into a glass and serve immediately.

Nutritional Value (per serving):

- **Calories:** 250
- **Total Fat:** 9g
- **Saturated Fat:** 7g
- **Cholesterol:** 0mg
- **Sodium:** 10mg
- **Total Carbohydrates**: 42g

- **Dietary Fiber:** 5g
- **Sugars:** 24g
- **Protein:** 2g

Cooking Tips:

- Use ripe bananas for natural sweetness and creaminess in the smoothie.
- For a thicker smoothie, use frozen banana chunks and pineapple chunks.
- Adjust the amount of honey or maple syrup according to your taste preferences.
- Fresh turmeric can be used instead of ground turmeric for added flavor and nutritional benefits.
- Add a splash of lemon juice for a citrusy twist to the smoothie.

Health Benefits:

1. **Anti-Inflammatory Properties:** Turmeric and ginger are both potent anti-inflammatory ingredients that may help reduce inflammation in the body, making this smoothie beneficial for individuals with inflammatory conditions such as arthritis or autoimmune diseases.
2. **Digestive Support:** Ginger is known for its digestive benefits, helping to alleviate nausea, aid digestion, and soothe an upset stomach.
3. **Immune Boost:** The combination of turmeric and ginger provides immune-boosting properties, supporting the body's natural defense mechanisms and promoting overall health and wellness.
4. **Antioxidant-Rich:** Turmeric and pineapple are rich in antioxidants, which help protect the body against oxidative stress and free radical damage.
5. **Heart Health:** Coconut milk contains healthy fats that may support heart health by improving cholesterol levels and reducing the risk of heart disease.

AIP Breakfast Bowl

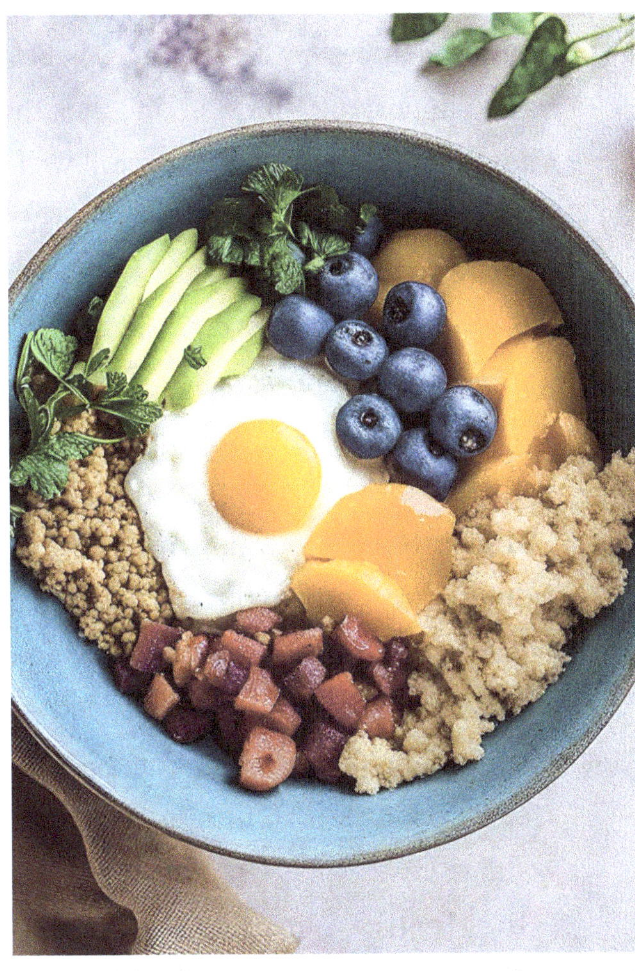

Time of Preparation: 15 minutes

Cooking Time: 10 minutes

Serving Units: 2

Ingredients:

- Two medium-sized peeled and diced sweet potatoes
- 1 tablespoon coconut oil
- 4 slices bacon, cooked and crumbled
- 2 cups baby spinach
- 1 avocado, sliced
- 4 poached eggs
- Salt and pepper to taste
- Fresh parsley for garnish (optional)

Procedures:

1. Place a skillet over medium heat and add the coconut oil. Add the cubed sweet potatoes and cook for 8-10 minutes, stirring occasionally, until they are tender and lightly browned.
2. While the sweet potatoes are cooking, poach the eggs in a separate pot of simmering water until the whites are set but the yolks are still runny, about 3-4 minutes.
3. Once the sweet potatoes are cooked, divide them between two serving bowls.
4. Top the sweet potatoes with baby spinach, crumbled bacon, sliced avocado, and poached eggs.
5. To taste, add salt and pepper for flavor.
6. Garnish with fresh parsley if desired.
7. Serve immediately and enjoy!

Nutritional Value (per serving):

- **Calories:** 450
- **Total Fat:** 30g
- **Saturated Fat:** 10g

- **Cholesterol:** 375mg
- **Sodium:** 380mg
- **Total Carbohydrates:** 30g
- **Dietary Fiber:** 9g
- **Sugars:** 6g
- **Protein:** 19g

Cooking Tips:

- Be sure to cube the sweet potatoes into small, evenly sized pieces to ensure they cook evenly and quickly.
- You can cook the bacon in advance and store it in the refrigerator until ready to use. Simply reheat it in the skillet before assembling the breakfast bowls.
- Feel free to customize the breakfast bowls with additional toppings such as sliced cherry tomatoes, sautéed mushrooms, or shredded chicken.
- If you prefer your eggs cooked differently, you can scramble or fry them instead of poaching.

Health Benefits:

1. **Nutrient-Rich:** This AIP Breakfast Bowl is packed with nutrient-dense ingredients such as sweet potatoes, spinach, avocado, and eggs, providing essential vitamins, minerals, and antioxidants to start your day on the right foot.
2. **Healthy Fats:** Avocado and coconut oil are sources of healthy fats, which are important for brain health, hormone production, and overall well-being.
3. **Protein-Packed:** Eggs and bacon are excellent sources of protein, helping to keep you full and satisfied until your next meal while supporting muscle repair and growth.
4. **Blood Sugar Regulation:** Sweet potatoes are a complex carbohydrate that provides sustained energy and helps regulate blood sugar levels, making this breakfast option suitable for individuals with insulin resistance or diabetes.
5. **Gut Health:** Spinach is rich in fiber, which supports digestive health and promotes a healthy gut microbiome. Additionally, the AIP diet emphasizes gut-healing foods, making this breakfast bowl beneficial for individuals with autoimmune diseases or digestive issues.

Sweet Potato Hash

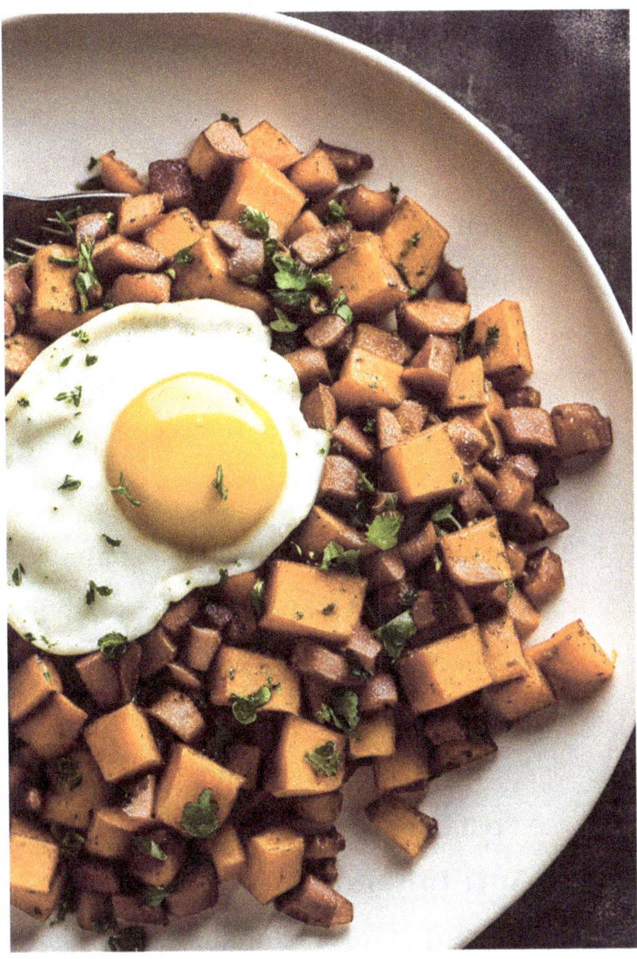

Time of Preparation: 10 minutes
Cooking Time: 20 minutes
Serving Units: 2

Ingredients:

- Two medium sweet potatoes, chopped into tiny pieces after peeling
- 1 tablespoon coconut oil or olive oil
- 1 small onion, diced
- 1 red bell pepper, diced
- 1 green bell pepper, diced
- 2 cloves garlic, minced
- 1 teaspoon ground paprika
- 1 teaspoon dried oregano
- Salt and pepper to taste
- 2-3 green onions, sliced (optional, for garnish)
- Fresh parsley, chopped (optional, for garnish)

Procedures:

1. Peel and dice the sweet potatoes into small, evenly sized cubes.
2. Heat the coconut oil or olive oil in a large skillet over medium heat.
3. Add the diced sweet potatoes to the skillet and cook for about 10 minutes, stirring occasionally, until they start to soften.
4. Add the diced onion, red bell pepper, and green bell pepper to the skillet. Continue to cook for another 7-8 minutes, stirring occasionally, until the vegetables are tender and the sweet potatoes are golden brown.
5. Add the minced garlic, ground paprika, and dried oregano to the skillet. Stir well to combine and cook for an additional 1-2 minutes until the garlic is fragrant.
6. Season with salt and pepper to taste.

7. Remove from heat and transfer the sweet potato hash to serving plates.

8. Garnish with sliced green onions and chopped fresh parsley if desired.

9. Serve immediately and enjoy!

Nutritional Value (per serving):

- **Calories:** 250
- **Total Fat:** 10g
- **Saturated Fat:** 7g
- **Cholesterol:** 0mg
- **Sodium:** 150mg
- **Total Carbohydrates:** 35g
- **Dietary Fiber:** 6g
- **Sugars:** 9g
- **Protein:** 3g

Cooking Tips:

- For even cooking, make sure to dice the sweet potatoes into small, uniform pieces.

- You can add other vegetables to the hash such as zucchini, mushrooms, or spinach for added variety and nutrition.

- If you prefer a bit of heat, add a pinch of cayenne pepper or red pepper flakes along with the other seasonings.

- To save time in the morning, you can peel and dice the sweet potatoes the night before and store them in an airtight container in the refrigerator.

- This hash pairs well with a protein source such as fried or poached eggs, grilled chicken, or sausage for a more substantial meal.

Health Benefits:

1. **Rich in Vitamins and Minerals:** Sweet potatoes are an excellent source of vitamins A and C, manganese, and potassium, which are essential for immune function, skin health, and muscle function.

2. **High in Fiber:** The fiber content in sweet potatoes and bell peppers helps support digestive health, promotes regularity, and aids in maintaining a healthy weight by keeping you full and satisfied.

3. **Anti-Inflammatory Properties:** Sweet potatoes contain antioxidants such as beta-carotene and vitamin C, which have anti-inflammatory properties that can help reduce inflammation and oxidative stress in the body.

4. **Heart Health:** The combination of fiber, potassium, and antioxidants in sweet potatoes and bell peppers supports heart health by regulating blood pressure and reducing the risk of cardiovascular diseases.

Coconut Flour Pancakes

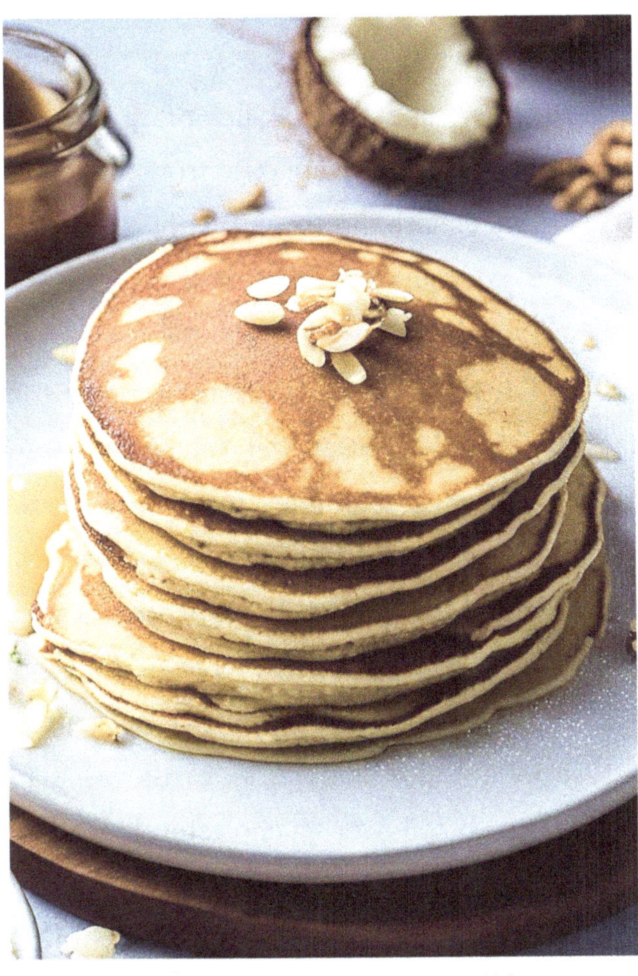

Time of Preparation: 10 minutes

Cooking Time: 15 minutes

Serving Units: 2-3 (makes about 6-8 small pancakes)

Ingredients:

- 1/4 cup coconut flour
- 1/2 teaspoon baking soda
- 1/4 teaspoon sea salt
- 4 large eggs
- 1/4 cup coconut milk (or any dairy-free milk of choice)
- One tablespoon (optional, for sweetness) of honey or maple syrup
- 1 teaspoon vanilla extract
- Coconut oil or ghee for cooking

Procedures:

1. In a medium bowl, combine the coconut flour, baking soda, and sea salt. Whisk to blend well.
2. In another bowl, whisk together the eggs, coconut milk, honey or maple syrup (if using), and vanilla extract until smooth.
3. Gradually add the wet ingredients to the dry ingredients, stirring until a smooth batter forms. Let the batter sit for a few minutes to allow the coconut flour to absorb the liquid and thicken slightly.
4. Add a little quantity of ghee or coconut oil to a non-stick pan or griddle and heat it over medium heat.
5. Pour about 2-3 tablespoons of batter onto the skillet for each pancake. Use the back of a spoon to spread the batter out into a small circle.
6. Cook the pancakes for 2-3 minutes on each side, or until bubbles form on the surface and the edges start to set.

After flipping, cook for a further two to three minutes, or until cooked through and golden brown.

7. Repeat with the remaining batter, adding more coconut oil or ghee to the skillet as needed.

8. Serve the pancakes warm with your favorite toppings such as fresh berries, sliced bananas, coconut yogurt, or a drizzle of honey or maple syrup.

Nutritional Value (per serving - approximately 3 pancakes):

- **Calories:** 220
- **Total Fat:** 15g
- **Saturated Fat:** 8g
- **Cholesterol:** 220mg
- **Sodium:** 350mg
- **Total Carbohydrates:** 11g
- **Dietary Fiber:** 4g
- **Sugars:** 5g
- **Protein:** 8g

Cooking Tips:

- Allow the batter to rest for a few minutes before cooking to let the coconut flour fully absorb the liquids, resulting in a better texture.
- Keep the heat at medium to avoid burning the pancakes, as coconut flour can brown quickly.
- If the batter seems too thick, add a bit more coconut milk, one tablespoon at a time, until the desired consistency is reached.
- Use a non-stick skillet or griddle to prevent the pancakes from sticking, and ensure they cook evenly.

Health Benefits:

1. **Gluten-Free:** Coconut flour is naturally gluten-free, making these pancakes suitable for those with gluten intolerance or celiac disease.

2. **High in Fiber:** Coconut flour is rich in dietary fiber, which aids in digestion, helps maintain a healthy weight, and supports cardiovascular health by lowering cholesterol levels.

3. **Low in Carbohydrates:** These pancakes are lower in carbohydrates compared to traditional wheat-based pancakes, making them a good option for those following a low-carb or ketogenic diet.

4. **Rich in Healthy Fats:** The use of coconut milk and coconut oil provides beneficial medium-chain triglycerides (MCTs) that can boost energy, enhance fat burning, and support brain health.

Berry Smoothie Bowl

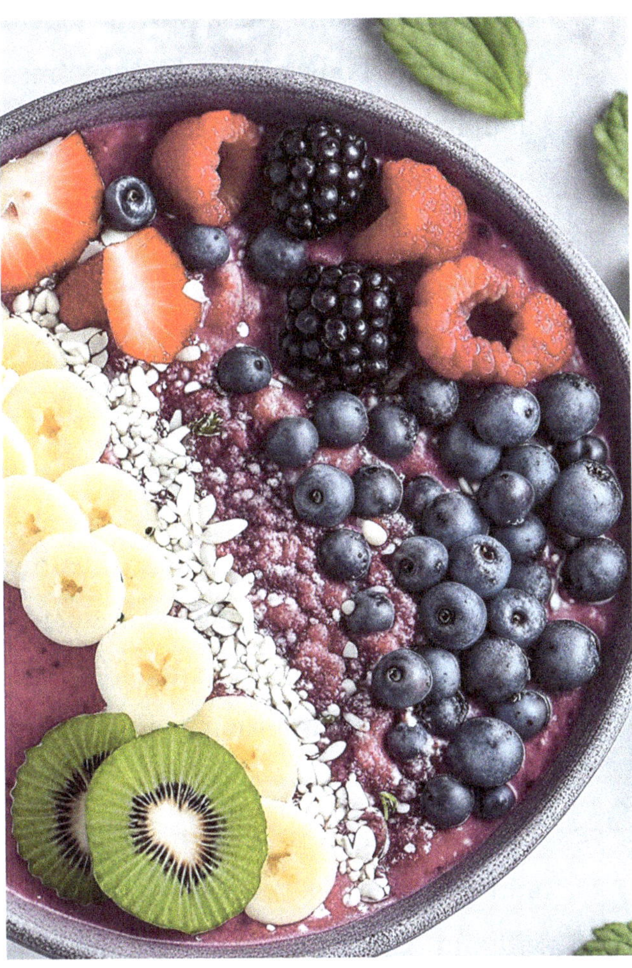

Time of Preparation: 10 minutes
Cooking Time: None
Serving Units: 1-2

Ingredients:

- One cup of mixed frozen berries, including blackberries, raspberries, blueberries, and strawberries
- 1 frozen banana
- 1/2 cup coconut milk (or any dairy-free milk of choice)
- One tablespoon (optional, for sweetness) of honey or maple syrup
- 1 teaspoon vanilla extract

Toppings:

- Fresh berries (blueberries, strawberries, raspberries)
- Sliced banana
- Shredded coconut
- Chia seeds
- Sliced almonds or other nuts/seeds
- Fresh mint leaves (optional)

Procedures:

1. In a blender, combine the frozen berries, frozen banana, coconut milk, honey or maple syrup (if using), and vanilla extract.
2. Process on high speed until creamy and smooth. If the mixture is too thick, add a bit more coconut milk, one tablespoon at a time, until the desired consistency is reached.
3. Pour the smoothie into a bowl.
4. Arrange your choice of toppings on the smoothie bowl. Popular options include fresh berries, sliced banana, shredded coconut, chia seeds, sliced almonds, and fresh mint leaves.

5. Serve immediately and enjoy!

Nutritional Value (per serving):

- **Calories:** 250
- **Total Fat:** 10g
- **Saturated Fat:** 7g
- **Cholesterol:** 0mg
- **Sodium:** 35mg
- **Total Carbohydrates:** 40g
- **Dietary Fiber:** 9g
- **Sugars:** 25g
- **Protein:** 3g

Cooking Tips:

- Use ripe, frozen bananas for a naturally sweet and creamy base.
- To make the smoothie thicker, use less liquid and ensure the fruit is fully frozen.
- Customize the smoothie bowl with your favorite toppings to add texture, flavor, and additional nutrients.
- If you don't have mixed berries, you can use a single type of berry or any combination you prefer.
- For added protein, you can blend in a scoop of collagen peptides or protein powder compatible with the AIP diet.

Health Benefits:

1. **Rich in Antioxidants:** Berries are loaded with antioxidants, which help protect the body from oxidative stress and free radical damage, supporting overall health and longevity.
2. **High in Fiber:** The berries and banana provide a good amount of dietary fiber, aiding digestion, promoting regularity, and helping to maintain healthy blood sugar levels.
3. **Supports Heart Health:** Berries are known for their heart-healthy properties, including reducing inflammation, lowering blood pressure, and improving cholesterol levels.
4. **Boosts Immunity:** The vitamins and minerals in berries, particularly vitamin C, strengthen the immune system and enhance the body's ability to fight infections.
5. **Promotes Healthy Skin:** The antioxidants and vitamins in berries help maintain healthy skin by reducing inflammation, preventing oxidative damage, and promoting collagen production.

2

Nourishing Soups and Stews

Healing Bone Broth Soup

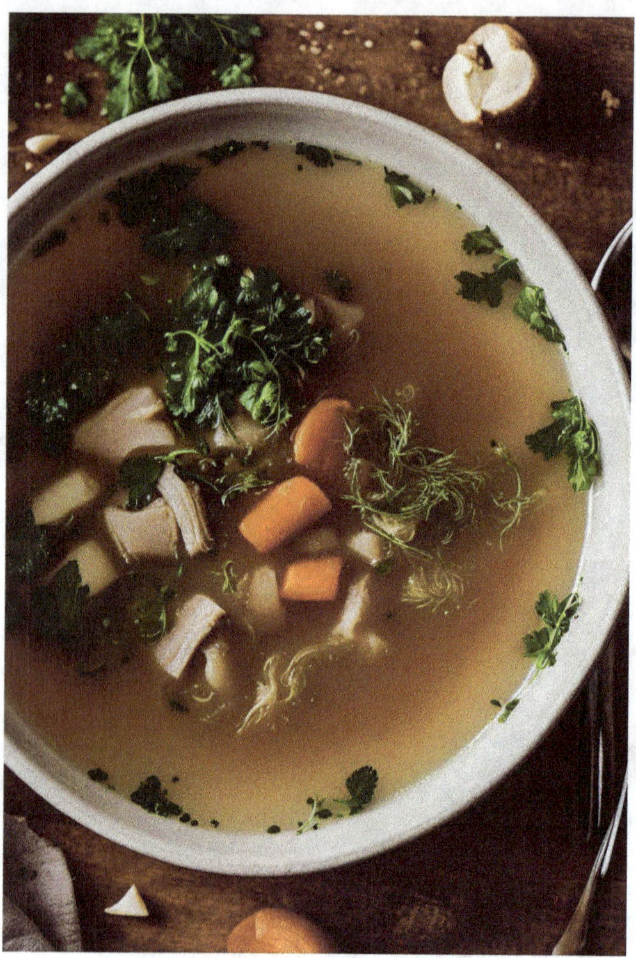

Time of Preparation: 20 minutes

Cooking Time: 4-24 hours (for simmering bone broth)

Serving Units: 4-6

Ingredients:

- 8 cups bone broth (homemade or store-bought)
- 2 cups cooked chicken, shredded or diced
- 2 carrots, peeled and sliced
- 2 celery stalks, sliced
- 1 onion, diced
- 3 cloves garlic, minced
- 1 tablespoon fresh ginger, grated
- 1 teaspoon ground turmeric
- 1 teaspoon dried thyme
- Salt and pepper to taste
- Fresh parsley, chopped (optional, for garnish)

Procedures:

1. In a large pot, bring the bone broth to a simmer over medium heat.
2. Add the cooked chicken, carrots, celery, onion, garlic, ginger, ground turmeric, and dried thyme to the pot.
3. To taste, add salt and pepper for seasoning.
4. Reduce the heat to low and let the soup simmer for at least 30 minutes to allow the flavors to meld together. For a richer flavor, simmer the soup for up to 4 hours or longer.
5. Once the vegetables are tender and the flavors have developed to your liking, remove the soup from heat.
6. Ladle the soup into serving bowls and garnish with fresh parsley if desired.
7. Serve hot and enjoy!

Nutritional Value (per serving):

- **Calories:** 150
- **Total Fat:** 5g
- **Saturated Fat:** 1.5g
- **Cholesterol:** 30mg
- **Sodium:** 600mg
- **Total Carbohydrates:** 10g
- **Dietary Fiber:** 2g
- **Sugars:** 3g
- **Protein:** 15g

Cooking Tips:

- Use homemade bone broth for the best flavor and nutritional value. You can make bone broth by simmering bones (such as chicken, beef, or turkey) with vegetables and herbs in water for several hours to extract the nutrients and collagen.
- If using store-bought bone broth, choose a high-quality, organic brand with no added preservatives or artificial ingredients.
- Feel free to customize the soup with additional vegetables such as diced potatoes, chopped kale, or sliced mushrooms.
- For a thicker soup, you can add a tablespoon of arrowroot powder or tapioca flour to thicken the broth.
- This soup can be made in advance and stored in the refrigerator for up to 3-4 days or frozen for longer storage. Before serving, gently reheat in the microwave or on the stove.

Health Benefits:

1. **Gut Health:** Bone broth is rich in gelatin and collagen, which are beneficial for gut health. They help repair the intestinal lining, reduce inflammation, and support digestive function.
2. **Joint Health:** The collagen and amino acids in bone broth help support joint health by promoting cartilage repair and reducing joint pain and inflammation.
3. **Immune Support:** The combination of nutrient-rich ingredients such as garlic, ginger, and turmeric, along with the immune-boosting properties of bone broth, makes this soup an excellent choice for supporting the immune system and warding off viruses and colds.
4. **Nutrient-Dense:** This soup is packed with vitamins, minerals, and antioxidants from the vegetables and herbs, providing essential nutrients for overall health and well-being.

Turmeric Chicken Soup

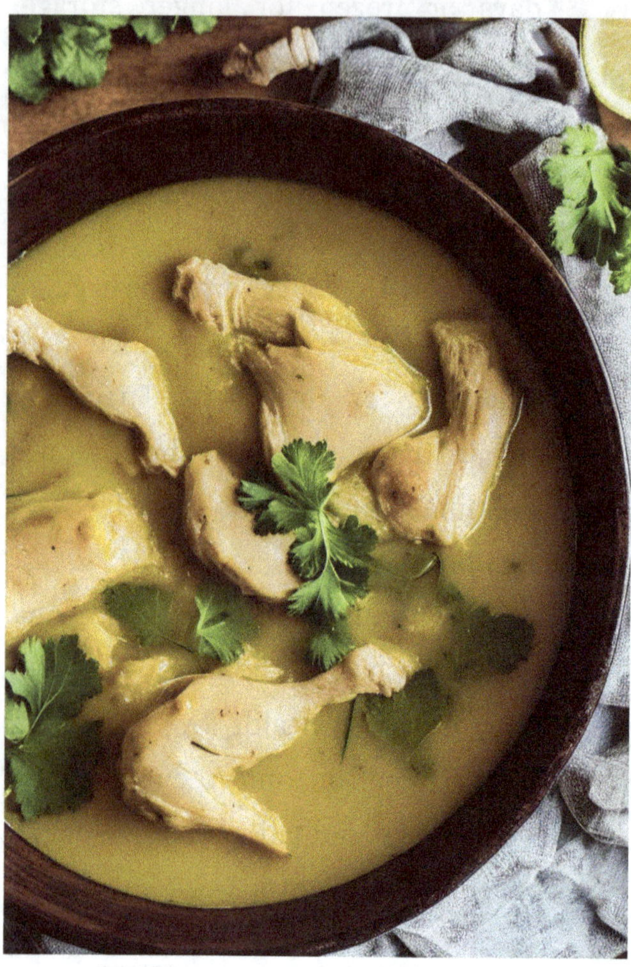

Time of Preparation: 15 minutes
Cooking Time: 30 minutes
Serving Units: 4-6

Ingredients:

- Two teaspoons of coconut oil or olive oil
- 1 medium onion, diced
- 3 cloves garlic, minced
- 1 tablespoon fresh ginger, grated
- 1 teaspoon ground turmeric
- 1 teaspoon ground cumin
- 1/2 teaspoon ground coriander
- 1/2 teaspoon ground black pepper
- 4 cups chicken broth (preferably homemade or low-sodium)
- 2 cups cooked, shredded chicken (about 2-3 chicken breasts)
- 2 large carrots, peeled and sliced
- 2 celery stalks, sliced
- 1 cup diced sweet potatoes (optional)
- 1 cup coconut milk (optional for creaminess)
- 2 cups baby spinach or kale, chopped
- Juice of 1 lemon
- Salt to taste
- Finely chopped fresh parsley or cilantro (optional for garnish)

Procedures:

1. In a large pot, heat the olive oil or coconut oil over medium heat.
2. Add the chopped onion and simmer for about 5 minutes, or until softened.
3. Cook the grated ginger and minced garlic for a further one to two minutes, or until fragrant.
4. Stir in the ground turmeric, cumin, coriander, and black pepper. Toast the spices for one minute.

5. Pour in the chicken broth and bring to a simmer.

6. Add the shredded chicken, carrots, celery, and sweet potatoes (if using). Simmer until the veggies are soft, approximately 20 minutes.

7. Stir in the coconut milk (if using) and cook for another 5 minutes.

8. Add the chopped spinach or kale and cook until wilted, about 2 minutes.

9. Stir in the lemon juice and season with salt to taste.

10. Remove from heat and ladle the soup into bowls.

11. Garnish with fresh cilantro or parsley if desired.

12. Serve hot and enjoy!

Cooking Tips:

- Use high-quality, organic chicken broth for the best flavor and nutritional benefits.
- For a heartier soup, you can add more vegetables such as diced zucchini, bell peppers, or peas.
- Adjust the amount of turmeric to your taste preference; start with 1 teaspoon and add more if you enjoy a stronger turmeric flavor.
- For added protein, consider including a can of drained and rinsed chickpeas.
- If you prefer a thicker soup, you can blend a portion of the soup with an immersion blender before adding the greens.

Nutritional Value (per serving):

- **Calories:** 250
- **Total Fat:** 15g
- **Saturated Fat:** 6g
- **Cholesterol:** 50mg
- **Sodium:** 400mg
- **Total Carbohydrates:** 15g
- **Dietary Fiber:** 3g
- **Sugars:** 5g
- **Protein:** 18g

Health Benefits:

1. **Anti-Inflammatory:** Turmeric contains curcumin, a powerful anti-inflammatory compound that helps reduce inflammation in the body and can be beneficial for those with arthritis, autoimmune diseases, or chronic pain.

2. **Immune Support:** This soup is packed with immune-boosting ingredients such as garlic, ginger, and turmeric, which help fight off

infections and support overall immune health.

3. **Digestive Health:** Ginger aids digestion and can help alleviate nausea, bloating, and indigestion. The fiber in vegetables like carrots and sweet potatoes also promotes healthy digestion.

4. **Rich in Nutrients:** The soup provides a good balance of protein from the chicken, healthy fats from the olive oil or coconut oil, and vitamins and minerals from the vegetables, making it a well-rounded meal.

5. **Bone Health:** Chicken broth made from bones is rich in collagen and minerals such as calcium and magnesium, which are essential for maintaining healthy bones and joints.

6. **Hydration and Detoxification:** The broth-based nature of the soup helps keep you hydrated, and the lemon juice adds a detoxifying effect by aiding in liver function and digestion.

Butternut Squash Soup

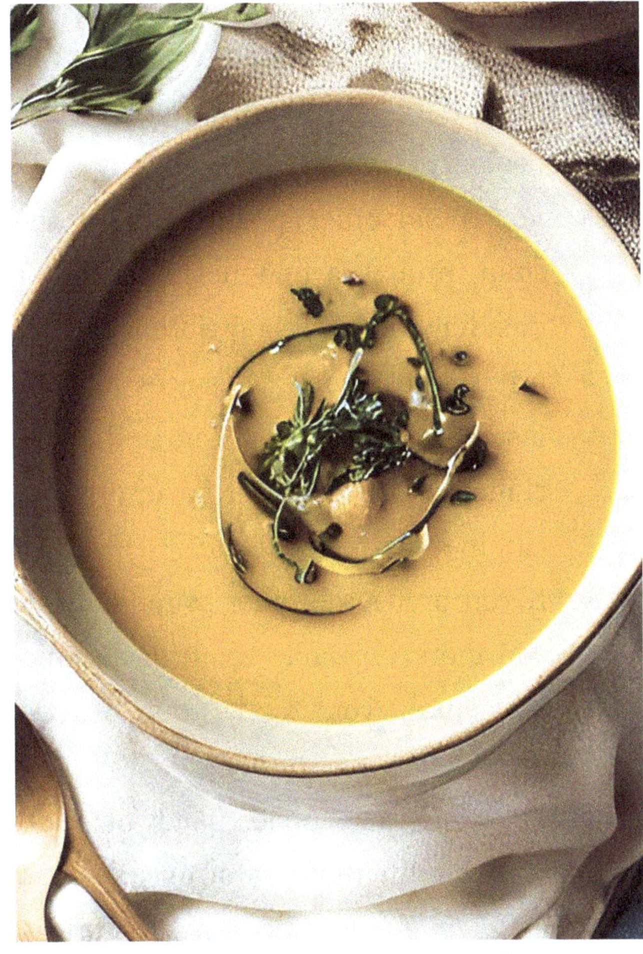

Time of Preparation: 15 minutes
Cooking Time: 45 minutes
Serving Units: 4-6

Ingredients:

- One big butternut squash, chopped, skinned, and seeded
- Two teaspoons of coconut oil or olive oil
- 1 onion, diced
- 2 cloves garlic, minced
- 1 teaspoon ground cumin
- 1/2 teaspoon ground cinnamon
- 1/4 teaspoon ground nutmeg
- 4 cups vegetable broth (preferably homemade or low-sodium)
- 1 cup coconut milk (or any dairy-free milk of choice)
- Salt and pepper to taste
- Fresh parsley or cilantro, chopped (optional, for garnish)

Procedures:

1. Preheat the oven to 400°F (200°C).
2. Place the diced butternut squash on a baking sheet lined with parchment paper. Drizzle with 1 tablespoon of olive oil or coconut oil and toss to coat evenly.
3. Roast the butternut squash in the preheated oven for 30-35 minutes, or until tender and lightly caramelized.
4. In a large pot, heat the remaining tablespoon of olive oil or coconut oil over medium heat.
5. Add the diced onion and cook until softened, about 5 minutes.
6. Add the minced garlic, ground cumin, ground cinnamon, and ground nutmeg to the pot. Cook until aromatic, one or two more minutes.

7. Add the roasted butternut squash to the pot and stir to combine with the onions and spices.

8. Pour in the vegetable broth and bring to a simmer. To enable the flavors to mingle together, boil the soup for around ten minutes.

9. Use an immersion blender to puree the soup until smooth and creamy. Or, you may move the soup, batch by batch, into a blender and process it until it's smooth, then pour it back into the pot.

10. Stir in the coconut milk and season with salt and pepper to taste.

11. Continue to cook the soup for another 5 minutes, stirring occasionally.

12. Remove from heat and ladle the soup into bowls.

13. If preferred, garnish with fresh cilantro or parsley.

14. Serve hot and enjoy!

Nutritional Value (per serving):

- **Calories:** 200
- **Total Fat:** 12g
- **Saturated Fat:** 8g
- **Cholesterol:** 0mg
- **Sodium:** 400mg
- **Total Carbohydrates:** 20g
- **Dietary Fiber:** 5g
- **Sugars:** 5g
- Protein: 3g

Cooking Tips:

- To make peeling and cutting the butternut squash easier, you can microwave it for 2-3 minutes before peeling to soften the skin slightly.

- For a smoother texture, strain the soup through a fine-mesh sieve after blending to remove any fibrous bits.

- Adjust the amount of spices to your taste preference; you can add more cinnamon for a sweeter flavor or more cumin for a smokier taste.

- If you prefer a thinner soup, you can add more vegetable broth or coconut milk until you reach your desired consistency.

- This soup can be made in advance and stored in the refrigerator for up to 3-4 days or frozen for longer storage. Before serving, slowly reheat over the burner.

Health Benefits:

1. **Rich in Vitamins and Minerals:** Butternut squash is packed with vitamins A, C, and E, as well as potassium, magnesium, and other essential nutrients that support overall health and well-being.

2. **Immune Boost:** The combination of spices such as cinnamon, cumin, and nutmeg, along with the vitamins and minerals in butternut squash, helps strengthen the immune system and protect against infections.

3. **Heart Health:** The fiber, potassium, and antioxidants in butternut squash support heart health by lowering cholesterol levels, regulating blood pressure, and reducing the risk of heart disease.

4. **Digestive Support:** The fiber content in butternut squash aids digestion, promotes regularity, and supports a healthy gut microbiome.

5. **Anti-Inflammatory:** The antioxidants and phytonutrients in butternut squash have anti-inflammatory properties, helping to reduce inflammation in the body and alleviate symptoms of inflammatory conditions such as arthritis or autoimmune diseases.

AIP Vegetable Stew

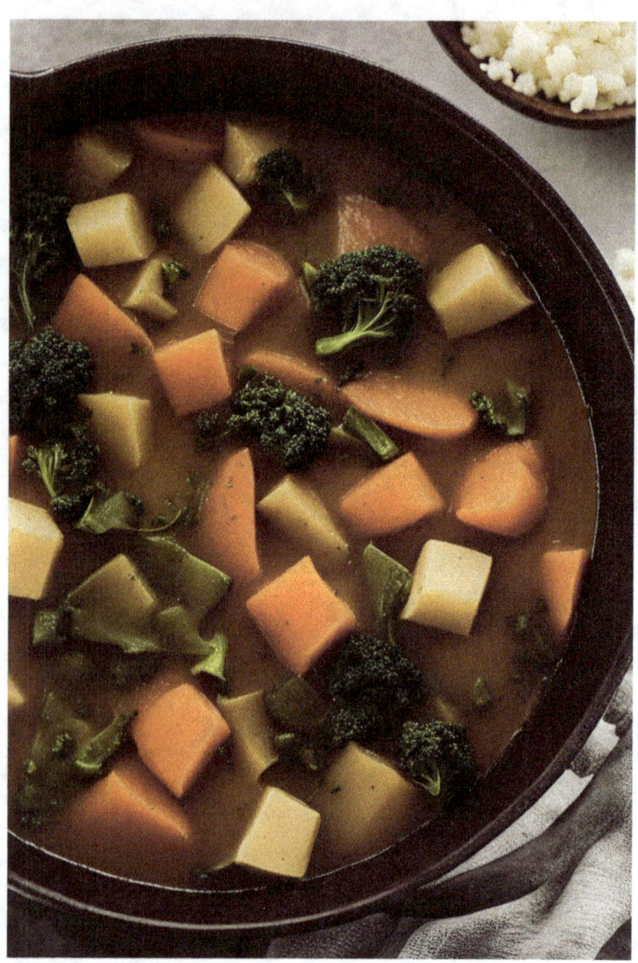

Time of Preparation: 20 minutes
Cooking Time: 40 minutes
Serving Units: 4-6

Ingredients:

- Two teaspoons of coconut oil or olive oil
- 1 large onion, diced
- 3 cloves garlic, minced
- 2 large carrots, peeled and sliced
- 2 celery stalks, sliced
- Diced and peeled sweet potato, big
- 1 cup butternut squash, peeled and diced
- 1 zucchini, diced
- One cup of cleaned and quartered green beans
- 1 can (14.5 oz) diced tomatoes (ensure AIP compliant, or use fresh diced tomatoes)
- 4 cups vegetable broth (preferably homemade or low-sodium)
- 1 teaspoon dried thyme
- 1 teaspoon dried oregano
- 1 teaspoon ground turmeric
- 1 bay leaf
- Salt to taste
- Chopped fresh parsley or cilantro (optional garnish)

Procedures:

1. Heat the olive oil or coconut oil in a large pot over medium heat.
2. Add the chopped onion and simmer for about 5 minutes, or until softened.
3. Add the minced garlic and stir until fragrant, another one to two minutes.
4. Add the sliced carrots, celery, sweet potato, butternut squash, zucchini, and green beans to the pot. After combining, cook for five minutes.

5. Pour in the diced tomatoes and vegetable broth.

6. Stir in the dried thyme, dried oregano, ground turmeric, and bay leaf.

7. Simmer the stew for a short while before turning down the heat. Cover and let it simmer for 30-40 minutes, or until the vegetables are tender.

8. Remove the bay leaf and season the stew with salt to taste.

9. Ladle the stew into bowls and garnish with fresh parsley or cilantro if desired.

10. Serve hot and enjoy!

Nutritional Value (per serving):

- **Calories:** 180
- **Total Fat:** 7g
- **Saturated Fat:** 1.5g
- **Cholesterol:** 0mg
- **Sodium:** 300mg
- **Total Carbohydrates:** 26g
- **Dietary Fiber:** 6g
- **Sugars:** 8g
- **Protein:** 4g

Cooking Tips:

- For a heartier stew, add a protein source such as diced chicken, turkey, or beef. Ensure the meat is AIP compliant and cooked before adding to the stew.

- Adjust the vegetables according to seasonality and personal preference. Other great additions include kale, spinach, or mushrooms.

- If you prefer a thicker stew, mash a few pieces of the sweet potato and butternut squash with a fork and stir them back into the stew.

- Ensure all ingredients, especially canned tomatoes, are free from additives and preservatives to remain AIP compliant.

- This stew can be made ahead and stored in the refrigerator for up to 4 days or frozen for longer storage. Before serving, slowly reheat over the burner.

Health Benefits:

1. **Rich in Vitamins and Minerals:** This vegetable stew is packed with a variety of vegetables, providing a wide range of essential vitamins and minerals such as vitamins A, C, K, potassium, and magnesium.

2. **Anti-Inflammatory:** Ingredients like turmeric and garlic have strong anti-inflammatory properties that help reduce inflammation in the body,

which is beneficial for those with autoimmune conditions.

3. **Digestive Health:** The fiber content from the vegetable's aids in digestion, promotes regular bowel movements, and supports a healthy gut microbiome.

4. **Immune Support:** The nutrient-dense vegetables and herbs in the stew, such as carrots, sweet potatoes, and thyme, help boost the immune system and protect against infections.

5. **Low in Calories and Fat:** This stew is a nutrient-dense, low-calorie, and low-fat meal, making it an excellent choice for maintaining a healthy weight and supporting overall well-being.

3

Satisfying Salads

Avocado Chicken Salad

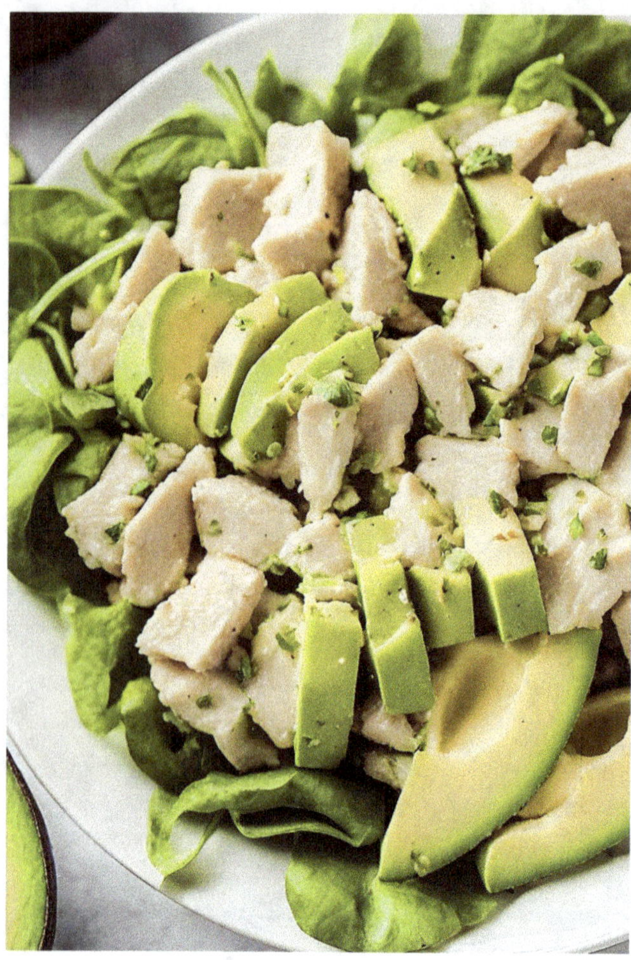

Time of Preparation: 15 minutes

Cooking Time: 15 minutes (for cooking chicken, if not using precooked chicken)

Serving Units: 4

Ingredients:

- Two cups cooked, chopped or shredded chicken breast
- 2 ripe avocados, peeled, pitted, and diced
- 1/2 cup red onion, finely chopped
- 1/2 cup cherry tomatoes, halved
- 1/4 cup cilantro or parsley, chopped
- Juice of 1 lime
- Salt and pepper to taste

For the Dressing:

- 1/4 cup plain Greek yogurt or dairy-free yogurt
- One spoonful of avocado or olive oil
- 1 tablespoon lime juice
- One teaspoon (optional, for sweetness) of honey or maple syrup
- 1/2 teaspoon garlic powder
- Salt and pepper to taste

Procedures:

1. In a large bowl, combine the cooked chicken, diced avocado, chopped red onion, cherry tomatoes, and chopped cilantro or parsley.

2. In a small bowl, whisk together the Greek yogurt, olive oil, lime juice, honey or maple syrup (if using), garlic powder, salt, and pepper to make the dressing.

3. Pour the dressing over the chicken and avocado mixture and toss gently to coat everything evenly.

4. Squeeze fresh lime juice over the salad and season with additional salt and pepper to taste, if needed.

5. Serve immediately, or refrigerate for 30 minutes to allow the flavors to meld together before serving.

6. Garnish with extra cilantro or parsley if desired.

Nutritional Value (per serving):

- **Calories:** 280
- **Total Fat:** 17g
- **Saturated Fat:** 3g
- **Cholesterol:** 70mg
- **Sodium:** 120mg
- **Total Carbohydrates:** 10g
- **Dietary Fiber:** 6g
- **Sugars:** 2g
- **Protein:** 25g

Cooking Tips:

- Use cooked chicken breast, either grilled, baked, or boiled, and shred or dice it as per your preference. Alternatively, you can use rotisserie chicken for added convenience.

- Make sure the avocados are ripe but still firm enough to hold their shape when diced.

- Tailor the lime juice quantity to your own desire. You can also add a pinch of cayenne pepper for extra heat if desired.

- To prevent the avocados from browning, toss them with lime juice as soon as they are diced and keep the salad covered until ready to serve.

- Customize the salad with additional ingredients such as diced bell peppers, cucumber, or black beans for extra flavor and texture.

Health Benefits:

1. **Healthy Fats:** Avocados are rich in heart-healthy monounsaturated fats, which help lower bad cholesterol levels, reduce the risk of heart disease, and support brain health.

2. **Fiber-Rich:** Avocados and vegetables in the salad provide dietary fiber, which aids digestion, promotes satiety, and supports a healthy gut microbiome.

3. **Vitamins and Minerals:** This salad is packed with vitamins and minerals from the chicken, avocado, and vegetables, including vitamin C, vitamin K, potassium, and folate, which are essential for overall health and well-being.

Roasted Beet and Arugula Salad

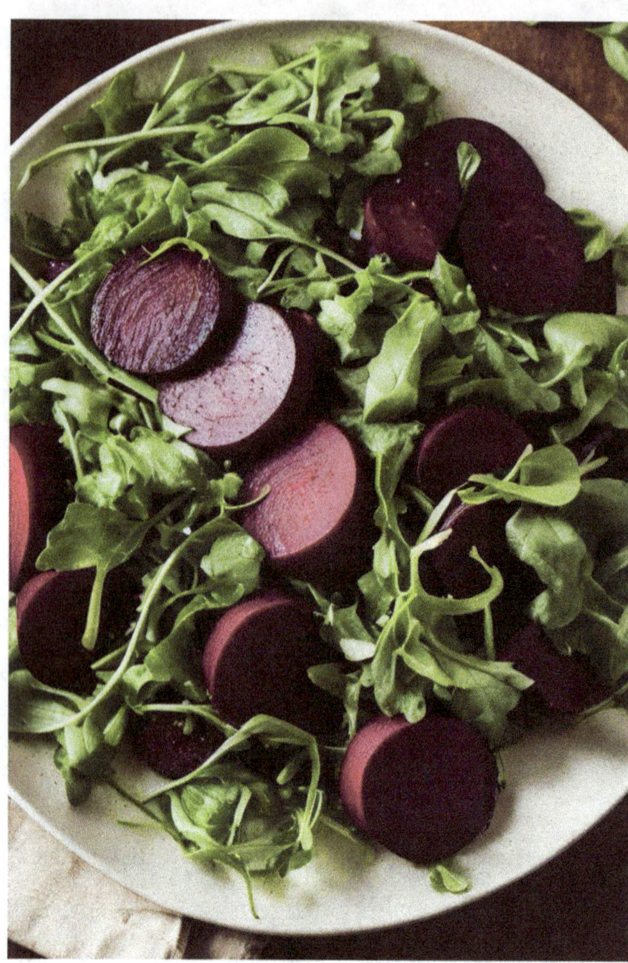

Time of Preparation: 15 minutes
Cooking Time: 45 minutes
Serving Units: 4

Ingredients:

- 3 medium beets, peeled and diced
- 2 tablespoons olive oil
- Salt and pepper to taste
- 4 cups fresh arugula
- 1/4 cup of optionally shredded feta or goat cheese
- 1/4 cup chopped pecans or walnuts (optional)
- A vinaigrette dressing or balsamic glaze to drizzle

Procedures:

1. Preheat the oven to 400°F (200°C).
2. Place the diced beets on a baking sheet lined with parchment paper.
3. Drizzle the beets with olive oil and season with salt and pepper to taste. Toss to coat evenly.
4. Roast the beets in the preheated oven for 30-35 minutes, or until tender and caramelized, stirring halfway through.
5. Remove the roasted beets from the oven and let them cool slightly.
6. In a large bowl, combine the fresh arugula with the roasted beets.
7. If using, sprinkle the crumbled goat cheese or feta cheese and chopped walnuts or pecans over the salad.
8. Drizzle the salad with balsamic glaze or vinaigrette dressing.
9. Toss gently to combine all the ingredients.
10. Serve immediately and enjoy!

Nutritional Value (per serving):

- **Calories:** 150
- **Total Fat:** 10g
- **Saturated Fat:** 2g
- **Cholesterol:** 5mg
- **Sodium:** 150mg
- **Total Carbohydrates:** 12g
- **Dietary Fiber:** 4g
- **Sugars:** 8g
- **Protein:** 4g

Cooking Tips:

- Choose beets that are firm and have smooth skin for the best flavor and texture.
- To make peeling beets easier, you can boil them for a few minutes before peeling or use a vegetable peeler.
- For a more intense flavor, you can roast the beets with herbs like thyme or rosemary.
- If you prefer a vegan option, you can omit the cheese or use a dairy-free alternative.
- Toast the walnuts or pecans in a dry skillet over medium heat for a few minutes to enhance their flavor before adding them to the salad.

Health Benefits:

1. **Rich in Antioxidants:** Beets are packed with antioxidants such as betalains and vitamin C, which help reduce inflammation, protect against oxidative stress, and support overall health.
2. **Heart Health:** The nitrates in beets help lower blood pressure, improve blood flow, and enhance cardiovascular health.
3. **Digestive Support:** Beets are high in dietary fiber, which promotes healthy digestion, regulates bowel movements, and supports gut health.
4. **Nutrient-Dense:** Arugula is rich in vitamins A, C, and K, as well as folate, calcium, and magnesium, providing essential nutrients for overall health and well-being.
5. **Bone Health:** Arugula contains vitamin K, which is important for bone health and helps prevent osteoporosis.
6. **Weight Management:** Arugula is low in calories and carbohydrates but high in fiber, making it a great choice for those looking to manage their weight or support weight loss goals.

Spinach and Strawberry Salad

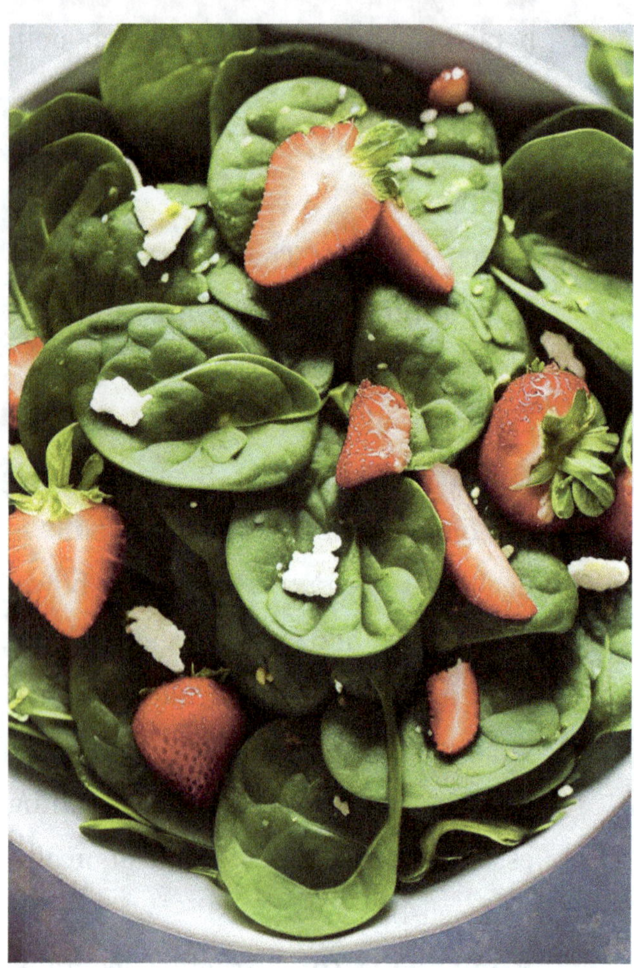

Time of Preparation: 15 minutes
Cooking Time: 0 minutes
Serving Units: 4

Ingredients:

- 6 cups fresh baby spinach leaves
- 1 1/2 cups fresh strawberries, sliced
- 1/4 cup red onion, thinly sliced
- 1/4 cup crumbled feta cheese or goat cheese (optional)
- 1/4 cup sliced almonds or pecans, toasted
- Balsamic vinaigrette dressing, for drizzling

Procedures:

1. In a large salad bowl, combine the fresh baby spinach leaves, sliced strawberries, and thinly sliced red onion.
2. If using, sprinkle the crumbled feta cheese or goat cheese and sliced almonds or pecans over the salad.
3. Drizzle the salad with balsamic vinaigrette dressing.
4. Toss gently to combine all the ingredients.
5. Serve immediately and enjoy!

Nutritional Value (per serving):

- **Calories:** 120
- **Total Fat:** 8g
- **Saturated Fat:** 2g
- **Cholesterol:** 5mg
- **Sodium:** 150mg
- **Total Carbohydrates:** 10g
- **Dietary Fiber:** 3g
- **Sugars:** 5g
- **Protein:** 4g

Cooking Tips:

- Choose fresh, ripe strawberries for the best flavor and sweetness.
- To toast sliced almonds or pecans, spread them in a single layer on a baking sheet and bake in a preheated oven at 350°F (175°C) for 5-7 minutes, or until lightly golden and fragrant. Watch them closely to prevent burning.
- Customize the salad by adding other ingredients such as avocado slices, grilled chicken or tofu, or cooked quinoa for added protein and texture.
- For a vegan option, omit the cheese or use a dairy-free alternative.
- Make the salad dressing ahead of time and store it in the refrigerator for up to one week for quick and easy meal prep.

Health Benefits:

1. **Rich in Antioxidants:** Spinach is packed with antioxidants such as vitamin C, vitamin E, and beta-carotene, which help protect cells from damage caused by free radicals, reduce inflammation, and support overall health.
2. **Heart Health:** Strawberries are rich in flavonoids and potassium, which help lower blood pressure, improve blood flow, and reduce the risk of heart disease.
3. **Bone Health:** Spinach is an excellent source of vitamin K, which is important for bone health and helps prevent osteoporosis.
4. **Weight Management:** Spinach is low in calories and carbohydrates but high in fiber, making it a great choice for those looking to manage their weight or support weight loss goals.
5. **Digestive Support:** The fiber content in spinach and strawberries aids in digestion, promotes regular bowel movements, and supports a healthy gut microbiome.
6. **Skin Health:** The vitamin C in strawberries helps promote collagen production, which is important for maintaining healthy skin, reducing wrinkles, and preventing premature aging.

Kale and Chicken Caesar Salad with Avocado Dressing

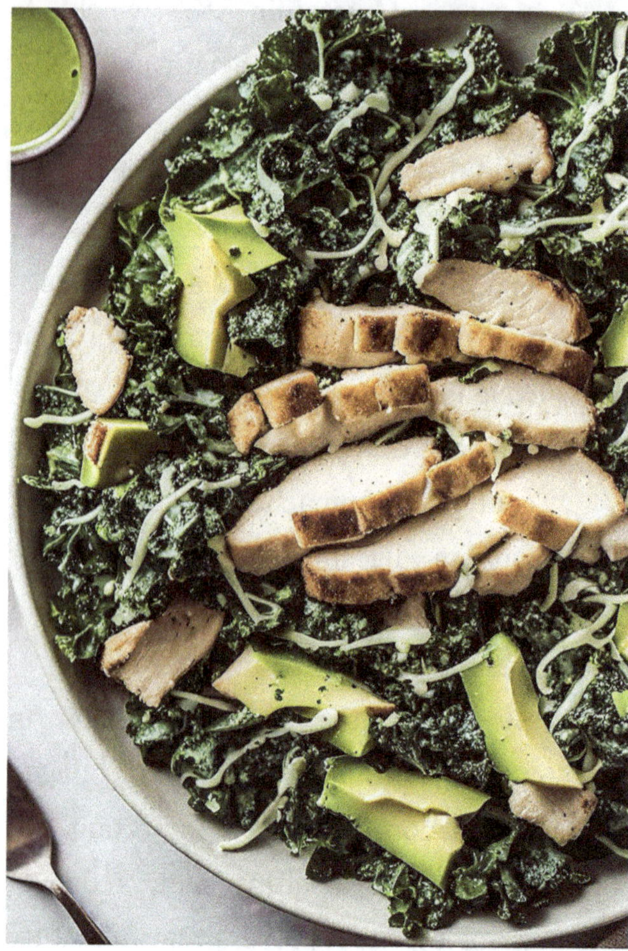

Time of Preparation: 20 minutes

Cooking Time: 15 minutes (for cooking chicken, if not using precooked chicken)

Serving Units: 4

Ingredients:

- One bunch of kale, shredded into bite-sized pieces with the stems removed
- Two cups cooked, chopped or shredded chicken breast
- 1 cup cherry tomatoes, halved
- 1/4 cup grated Parmesan cheese (optional)
- 1/4 cup croutons (optional)

For the Avocado Dressing:

- 1 ripe avocado, peeled and pitted
- 1/4 cup plain Greek yogurt or dairy-free yogurt
- 2 tablespoons olive oil
- 2 tablespoons fresh lemon juice
- 1 clove garlic, minced
- Salt and pepper to taste

Procedures:

1. In a large salad bowl, combine the torn kale leaves, cooked chicken breast, and cherry tomatoes.
2. In a blender or food processor, combine the avocado, Greek yogurt, olive oil, lemon juice, minced garlic, salt, and pepper.
3. Blend until smooth and creamy, adding a splash of water if needed to reach your desired consistency.
4. Pour the avocado dressing over the salad and toss gently to coat all the ingredients evenly.

5. If using, sprinkle the grated Parmesan cheese and croutons over the salad.

6. Serve immediately and enjoy!

Nutritional Value (per serving):

- **Calories:** 280
- **Total Fat:** 18g
- **Saturated Fat:** 3g
- **Cholesterol:** 70mg
- **Sodium:** 200mg
- **Total Carbohydrates:** 12g
- **Dietary Fiber:** 5g
- **Sugars:** 3g
- **Protein:** 22g

Cooking Tips:

- Massage the kale leaves with a little olive oil and lemon juice before assembling the salad to help soften them and improve their texture.
- Customize the salad by adding other ingredients such as sliced avocado, hard-boiled eggs, or bacon for added flavor and texture.
- For a vegan option, omit the chicken and cheese or use dairy-free alternatives.
- Use homemade croutons or choose whole-grain or gluten-free croutons for a healthier option.
- Double the recipe for the avocado dressing and store any leftovers in an airtight container in the refrigerator for up to three days for quick and easy meal prep.

Health Benefits:

1. **Nutrient-Dense Greens:** Kale is packed with vitamins A, C, and K, as well as minerals like calcium and potassium, providing essential nutrients for overall health and well-being.

2. **Healthy Fats:** Avocado is rich in heart-healthy monounsaturated fats, which help lower bad cholesterol levels, reduce the risk of heart disease, and support brain health.

3. **Antioxidants:** Cherry tomatoes are rich in antioxidants such as lycopene and vitamin C, which help protect cells from damage caused by free radicals, reduce inflammation, and support overall health.

4. **Bone Health:** Kale is an excellent source of vitamin K, which is important for bone health and helps prevent osteoporosis.

5. **Digestive Support:** The fiber content in kale and avocado aids in digestion, promotes regular bowel movements, and supports a healthy gut microbiome.

4

Main and side Dishes

Herb-Crusted Salmon

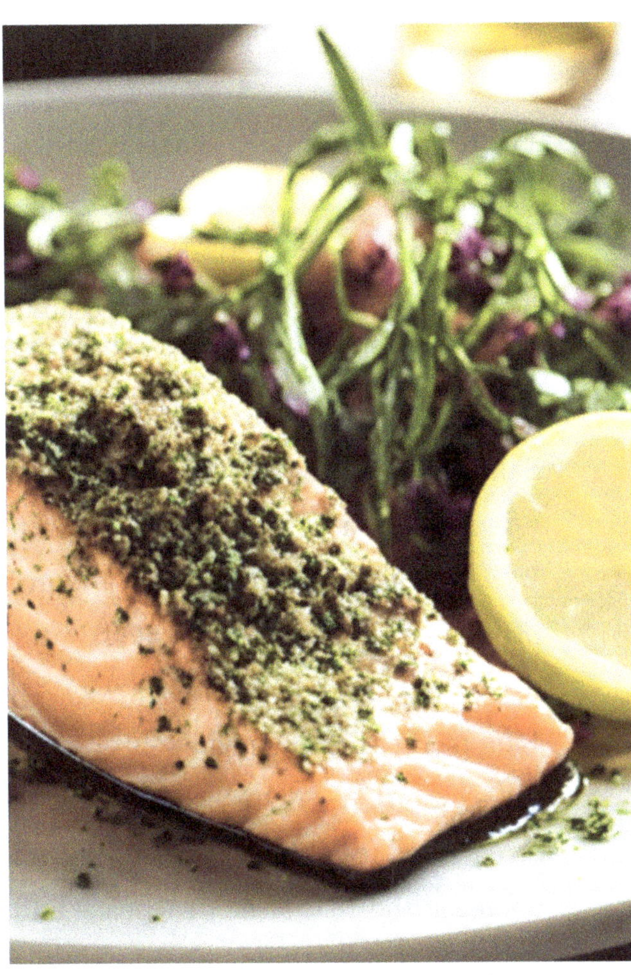

Time of Preparation: 10 minutes
Cooking Time: 15 minutes
Serving Units: 4

Ingredients:

- 4 salmon fillets, skin-on or skinless
- 2 tablespoons olive oil
- 2 tablespoons Dijon mustard
- 1/4 cup fresh herbs (such as parsley, dill, and thyme), finely chopped
- 1/4 cup almond flour or breadcrumbs (gluten-free if needed)
- Salt and pepper to taste
- Lemon wedges, for serving

Procedures:

1. Preheat the oven to 400°F (200°C). Line a baking sheet with parchment paper.
2. In a small bowl, mix together the olive oil and Dijon mustard.
3. In another bowl, combine the chopped herbs with almond flour or breadcrumbs.
4. Pat the salmon fillets dry with paper towels and season both sides with salt and pepper.
5. Brush the top of each salmon fillet with the olive oil and mustard mixture.
6. Press the herb and almond flour or breadcrumb mixture onto the top of each salmon fillet, covering it evenly.
7. Place the coated salmon fillets on the prepared baking sheet.
8. Bake in the preheated oven for 12-15 minutes, or until the salmon is cooked through and flakes easily with a fork.
9. Remove from the oven and let the salmon rest for a few minutes before serving.

10. Serve the herb-crusted salmon with lemon wedges on the side.

overcooking. With a fork, the salmon should flake easily and be opaque.

Nutritional Value (per serving):

- **Calories:** 300
- **Total Fat:** 18g
- **Saturated Fat:** 3g
- **Cholesterol:** 80mg
- **Sodium:** 200mg
- **Total Carbohydrates:** 2g
- **Dietary Fiber:** 1g
- **Sugars:** 0g
- **Protein:** 30g

Cooking Tips:

- Make sure the salmon fillets are evenly coated with the olive oil and mustard mixture to help the herb and almond flour or breadcrumb mixture adhere to them.
- To achieve the finest flavor, use a variety of fresh herbs. You can also use dried herbs if fresh ones are not available, but adjust the quantities accordingly.
- If using skin-on salmon fillets, place them skin-side down on the baking sheet to ensure even cooking and a crispy crust.
- Check the salmon for doneness after 12 minutes of baking to prevent

Health Benefits:

1. **High in Omega-3 Fatty Acids:** Salmon is rich in omega-3 fatty acids, which are essential for brain health, heart health, and reducing inflammation in the body.
2. **Rich in Vitamins and Minerals:** Salmon is packed with vitamins and minerals such as vitamin D, vitamin B12, selenium, and potassium, providing essential nutrients for overall health and well-being.
3. **Heart Health:** Omega-3 fatty acids in salmon help lower triglyceride levels, reduce blood pressure, and decrease the risk of heart disease and stroke.
4. **Bone Health:** Vitamin D and calcium in salmon are important for bone health and help prevent osteoporosis and bone fractures.
5. **Antioxidants:** Fresh herbs like parsley, dill, and thyme are rich in antioxidants, which help protect cells from damage caused by free radicals, reduce inflammation, and support overall health.

Lemon Garlic Chicken Thighs

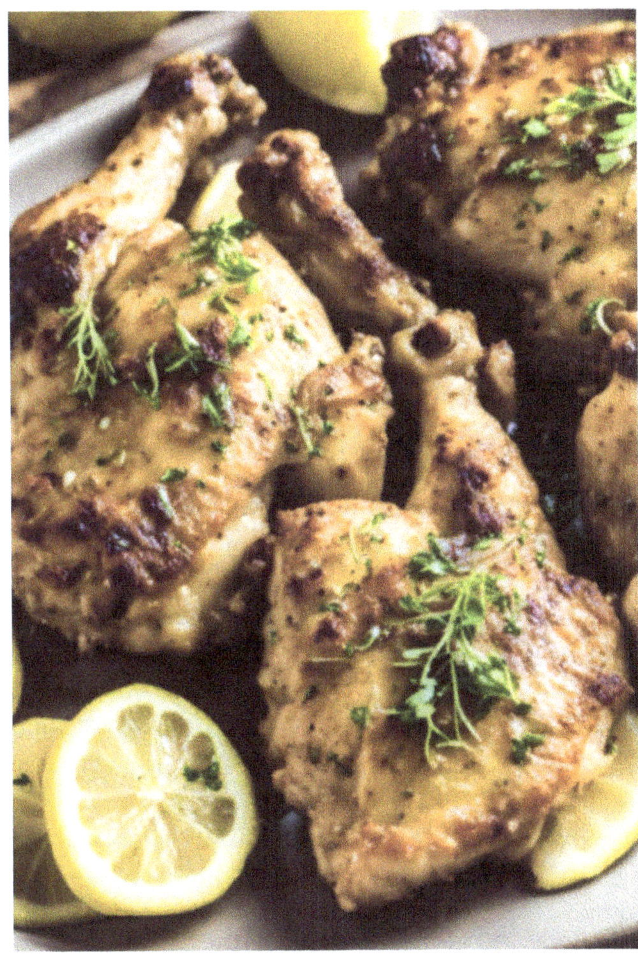

Time of Preparation: 10 minutes
Cooking Time: 25 minutes
Serving Units: 4

Ingredients:

- 8 bone-in, skin-on chicken thighs
- 4 cloves garlic, minced
- Zest of 1 lemon
- Juice of 2 lemons
- 2 tablespoons olive oil
- 2 teaspoons dried thyme
- Salt and pepper to taste
- Fresh parsley, chopped, for garnish

Procedures:

1. Preheat the oven to 400°F (200°C). Line a baking sheet with parchment paper.
2. In a small bowl, combine the minced garlic, lemon zest, lemon juice, olive oil, dried thyme, salt, and pepper.
3. Place the chicken thighs on the prepared baking sheet.
4. Brush the lemon garlic mixture over each chicken thigh, coating them evenly.
5. Bake in the preheated oven for 20-25 minutes, or until the chicken is cooked through and golden brown, with an internal temperature of 165°F (75°C).
6. Take the chicken out of the oven, and give it a few minutes to rest before serving.
7. Before serving, garnish with freshly cut parsley.

Nutritional Value (per serving):

- **Calories:** 350
- **Total Fat:** 25g
- **Saturated Fat:** 6g
- **Cholesterol:** 150mg

- **Sodium:** 200mg
- **Total Carbohydrates:** 2g
- **Dietary Fiber:** 0g
- **Sugars:** 0g
- **Protein:** 30g

Cooking Tips:

- If using boneless, skinless chicken thighs, reduce the cooking time slightly to prevent them from drying out.
- For extra crispy skin, you can sear the chicken thighs in a hot skillet for 2-3 minutes on each side before transferring them to the oven.
- Use fresh lemon juice for the best flavor, and reserve some lemon slices to garnish the chicken before serving.
- Make sure to evenly distribute the lemon garlic mixture over the chicken thighs to ensure they are well-coated and flavorful.
- Serve the lemon garlic chicken thighs with your favorite side dishes, such as roasted vegetables, mashed potatoes, or a fresh salad, for a complete and satisfying meal.

Health Benefits:

1. **High in Protein:** Chicken thighs are a rich source of protein, which is important for building and repairing tissues, supporting muscle growth, and keeping you feeling full and satisfied.
2. **Vitamin C:** Lemon juice is high in vitamin C, which supports a healthy immune system, promotes collagen production for healthy skin, and acts as an antioxidant to protect cells from damage caused by free radicals.
3. **Heart Health:** Olive oil used in the marinade is rich in heart-healthy monounsaturated fats, which help lower bad cholesterol levels, reduce the risk of heart disease, and support overall cardiovascular health.
4. **Antioxidants:** Garlic contains antioxidants that help reduce inflammation, lower blood pressure, and support cardiovascular health.
5. **Bone Health:** Chicken thighs are a good source of phosphorus and zinc, which are important for bone health and help prevent osteoporosis and bone fractures.
6. **Low in Carbohydrates:** This dish is low in carbohydrates and sugar, making it suitable for low-carb or ketogenic diets and helping to regulate blood sugar levels.

Turkey and Sweet Potato Skillet

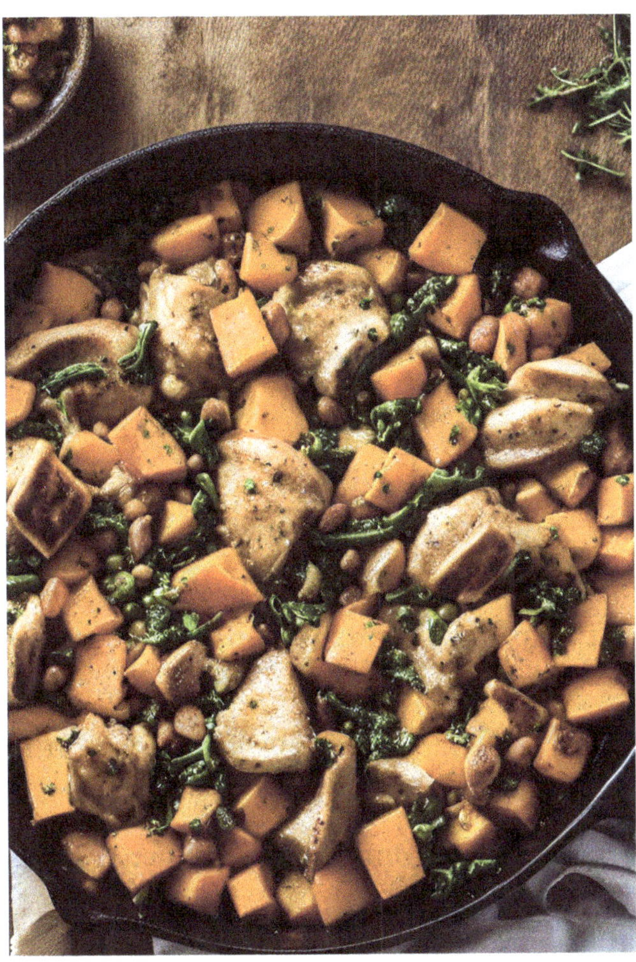

Time of Preparation: 15 minutes

Cooking Time: 25 minutes

Serving Units: 4

Ingredients:

- 1 lb. ground turkey
- Diced and peeled two medium sweet potatoes
- 1 onion, diced
- 2 cloves garlic, minced
- 1 bell pepper, diced (any color)
- 1 cup cherry tomatoes, halved
- 2 cups baby spinach
- 2 tablespoons olive oil
- 1 teaspoon paprika
- 1/2 teaspoon ground cumin
- Salt and pepper to taste
- Fresh parsley or cilantro, chopped, for garnish

Procedures:

1. In a big skillet over medium heat, warm up the olive oil.
2. Add diced sweet potatoes to the skillet and cook for about 5 minutes until they start to soften.
3. Add diced onion and minced garlic to the skillet and cook for another 2-3 minutes until fragrant.
4. Push the sweet potatoes, onion, and garlic to one side of the skillet and add ground turkey to the empty side.
5. Cook the ground turkey, breaking it up with a spatula, until it is browned and cooked through.
6. Mix the cooked turkey with the sweet potatoes, onion, and garlic in the skillet.
7. Add diced bell pepper, cherry tomatoes, paprika, ground cumin, salt, and pepper to the skillet.

8. Stir everything together and cook for another 5-7 minutes until the vegetables are tender and the flavors are well combined.

9. Add baby spinach to the skillet and cook for 2-3 minutes until wilted.

10. Remove the skillet from heat and garnish with chopped parsley or cilantro before serving.

Nutritional Value (per serving):

- **Calories:** 320
- **Total Fat:** 15g
- **Saturated Fat:** 3g
- **Cholesterol:** 60mg
- **Sodium:** 180mg
- **Total Carbohydrates:** 25g
- **Dietary Fiber:** 5g
- **Sugars:** 7g
- **Protein:** 22g

Cooking Tips:

- To save time, you can use pre-cooked or leftover sweet potatoes instead of cooking them from scratch in the skillet.
- Feel free to customize the recipe by adding your favorite vegetables such as zucchini, mushrooms, or corn.
- Adjust the seasoning according to your taste preference, adding more or less paprika, cumin, salt, and pepper as needed.
- For up to three to four days, keep any leftovers refrigerated in an airtight container. Before serving, gently reheat in the microwave or on the stove.

Health Benefits:

1. **Lean Protein:** Ground turkey is a lean source of protein, which is essential for muscle growth, repair, and overall body function.

2. **Complex Carbohydrates:** Sweet potatoes are a nutritious source of complex carbohydrates, providing sustained energy and supporting overall health.

3. **Antioxidants:** Bell peppers, cherry tomatoes, and spinach are rich in antioxidants such as vitamin C and beta-carotene, which help reduce inflammation, protect cells from damage caused by free radicals, and lower the risk of chronic diseases.

4. **Low in Sodium:** By using minimal added salt and relying on herbs and spices for flavor, this recipe is lower in sodium, making it suitable for those watching their sodium intake or managing hypertension.

Garlic and Herb Roasted Vegetables

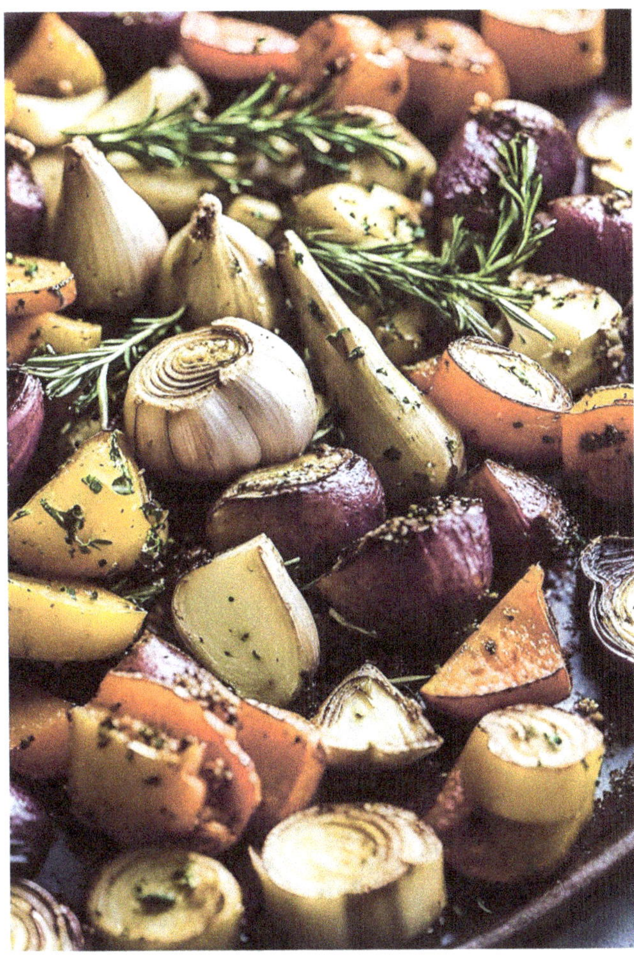

Time of Preparation: 15 minutes

Cooking Time: 25-30 minutes

Serving Units: 4

Ingredients:

- 1 lb mixed vegetables (such as carrots, potatoes, Brussels sprouts, bell peppers, and zucchini), washed and chopped into bite-sized pieces
- 3 cloves garlic, minced
- 2 tablespoons olive oil
- 1 teaspoon dried thyme
- 1 teaspoon dried rosemary
- Salt and pepper to taste
- Fresh parsley, chopped, for garnish (optional)

Procedures:

1. Preheat the oven to 425°F (220°C). For easier cleanup, line a baking pan with aluminum foil or parchment paper.
2. In a large bowl, combine the chopped mixed vegetables with minced garlic, olive oil, dried thyme, dried rosemary, salt, and pepper. Toss until the spice mixture coats the veggies evenly.
3. Spread the seasoned vegetables in a single layer on the prepared baking sheet, making sure they are not overcrowded. This enables them to caramelize on the outside and roast more evenly.
4. Roast the vegetables in the preheated oven for 25-30 minutes, or until they are tender and golden brown, stirring halfway through the cooking time for even browning.
5. Once the vegetables are roasted to perfection, remove them from the

oven and transfer them to a serving dish.

6. Garnish with chopped fresh parsley if desired, and serve immediately as a delicious and nutritious side dish or as a main course with grains or protein of your choice.

Nutritional Value (per serving):

- **Calories:** 120
- **Total Fat:** 7g
- **Saturated Fat:** 1g
- **Cholesterol:** 0mg
- **Sodium:** 30mg
- **Total Carbohydrates:** 14g
- **Dietary Fiber:** 4g
- **Sugars:** 4g
- **Protein:** 2g

Cooking Tips:

- Use a variety of colorful vegetables for visual appeal and a diverse range of flavors and nutrients. Experiment with different combinations based on your preferences and seasonal availability.
- To guarantee equal cooking, cut the veggies into uniform-sized pieces. While smaller portions could cook faster, larger ones might need to cook for longer periods of time.

- Don't overcrowd the baking sheet. Spread the vegetables in a single layer with some space between them to allow for proper air circulation and caramelization.
- For extra flavor, you can add additional herbs and spices such as oregano, thyme, rosemary, paprika, or cayenne pepper to the seasoning mixture.
- Serve the roasted vegetables immediately while they are hot and crispy for the best texture and flavor. Leftovers can be stored in an airtight container in the refrigerator for up to 3-4 days and reheated in the oven or microwave before serving.

Health Benefits:

1. **Nutrient-Rich:** Mixed vegetables are packed with essential vitamins, minerals, and antioxidants that are important for overall health and well-being. These include vitamin A, vitamin C, vitamin K, potassium, and folate, among others.
2. **Fiber:** Vegetables are high in dietary fiber, which promotes digestive health, regulates bowel movements, and helps maintain a healthy weight

by promoting satiety and reducing the risk of overeating.

3. **Antioxidants:** Garlic and herbs such as thyme and rosemary are rich in antioxidants, which help reduce inflammation, protect cells from damage caused by free radicals, and lower the risk of chronic diseases such as heart disease and cancer.

4. **Heart Health:** Olive oil used in the seasoning mixture is rich in heart-healthy monounsaturated fats, which help lower bad cholesterol levels, reduce the risk of heart disease, and support overall cardiovascular health.

5. **Low in Calories:** Roasted vegetables are naturally low in calories and fat, making them a nutritious and weight-friendly option for those looking to manage their calorie intake or lose weight.

6. **Versatile:** This recipe is highly customizable and adaptable to suit individual preferences and dietary restrictions. It can easily be made vegan, gluten-free, or dairy-free by using suitable ingredients and seasonings.

Cauliflower Rice Stir-Fry

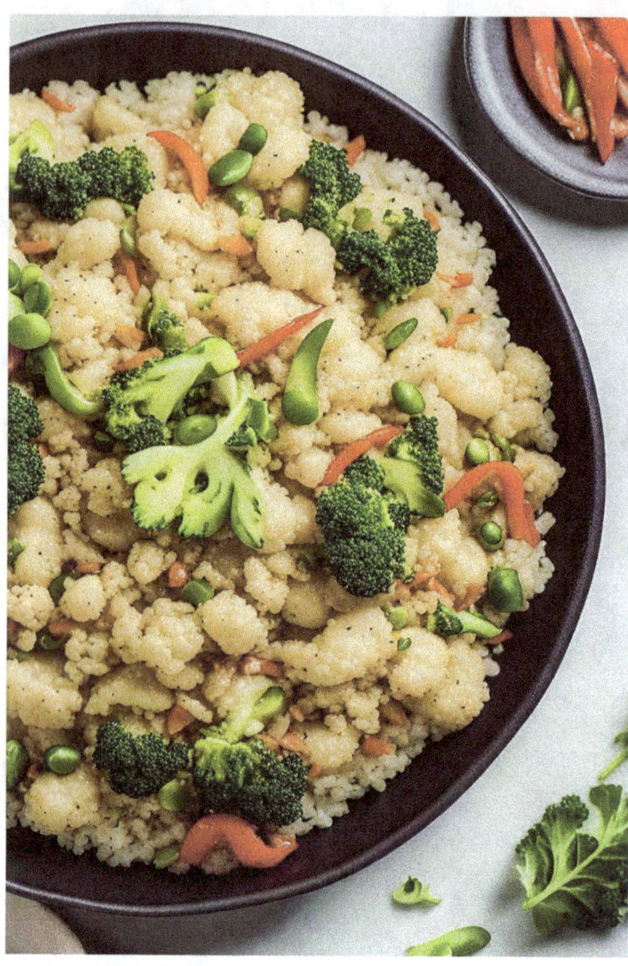

Time of Preparation: 15 minutes
Cooking Time: 10 minutes
Serving Units: 4

Ingredients:

- 1 medium head of cauliflower
- 2 tablespoons sesame oil or olive oil
- 3 cloves garlic, minced
- 1 onion, diced
- 2 carrots, diced
- 1 bell pepper, diced
- 1 cup broccoli florets
- One cup frozen pea, snow peas
- Two teaspoons of gluten-free tamari or soy sauce
- 1 tablespoon rice vinegar
- 1 teaspoon sriracha or chili paste (optional)
- Salt and pepper to taste
- For garnish, finely slice two green onions
- Sesame seeds, for garnish (optional)

Procedures:

1. Remove the leaves and stem from the cauliflower head, and chop the cauliflower into florets.
2. Place the cauliflower florets in a food processor and pulse until they resemble rice-like grains. Be careful not to over-process, as you want a rice-like texture, not a paste.
3. Heat sesame oil or olive oil in a large skillet or wok over medium heat.
4. Add minced garlic and diced onion to the skillet and sauté for 2-3 minutes until fragrant and translucent.
5. Add diced carrots, bell pepper, broccoli florets, and snap peas to the skillet and stir-fry for another 3-4

minutes until the vegetables are tender-crisp.

6. Push the vegetables to one side of the skillet and add the cauliflower rice to the empty side.

7. Pour soy sauce or tamari, rice vinegar, and sriracha or chili paste (if using) over the cauliflower rice.

8. Stir-fry the cauliflower rice for 3-4 minutes until it is heated through and slightly golden.

9. Mix the cauliflower rice with the stir-fried vegetables in the skillet until well combined.

10. Season with salt and pepper to taste, and garnish with thinly sliced green onions and sesame seeds before serving.

Nutritional Value (per serving):

- **Calories:** 120
- **Total Fat:** 6g
- **Saturated Fat:** 1g
- **Cholesterol:** 0mg
- **Sodium:** 400mg
- **Total Carbohydrates:** 15g
- **Dietary Fiber:** 6g
- **Sugars:** 6g
- **Protein:** 5g

Cooking Tips:

- Use a food processor to quickly and easily transform cauliflower florets into rice-like grains. As an alternative, you may shred the cauliflower into the rice using a box grater.

- Customize the stir-fry by adding your favorite vegetables such as mushrooms, cabbage, or baby corn.

- For added protein, you can stir in cooked tofu, chicken, shrimp, or beef to make it a complete meal.

- Adjust the seasoning and spiciness according to your taste preference by adding more or less soy sauce, rice vinegar, and sriracha or chili paste.

- Be careful not to overcook the vegetables, as you want them to retain their vibrant colors and crisp texture.

- Serve the cauliflower rice stir-fry as a flavorful and nutritious main course or as a side dish to complement your favorite protein.

Health Benefits:

1. **Low in Calories and Carbohydrates:** Cauliflower rice is a low-calorie and low-carbohydrate alternative to traditional rice, making it suitable for those watching their

calorie or carb intake or following a ketogenic diet.

2. **Rich in Fiber:** Cauliflower rice is high in dietary fiber, which promotes digestive health, regulates bowel movements, and helps keep you feeling full and satisfied.

3. **Vitamins and Minerals:** Cauliflower is packed with vitamins C and K, as well as folate, potassium, and manganese, providing essential nutrients for overall health and well-being.

4. **Antioxidants:** The colorful assortment of vegetables in this stir-fry is rich in antioxidants such as vitamin C, beta-carotene, and flavonoids, which help reduce inflammation, protect cells from damage caused by free radicals, and lower the risk of chronic diseases.

5. **Weight Management:** Cauliflower rice is low in calories and carbohydrates but high in fiber, making it a great choice for those looking to manage their weight or support weight loss goals.

6. **Gluten-Free and Paleo-Friendly:** This recipe is naturally gluten-free and paleo-friendly, making it suitable for those with gluten sensitivities or following a paleo diet.

Garlic Mashed Sweet Potatoes

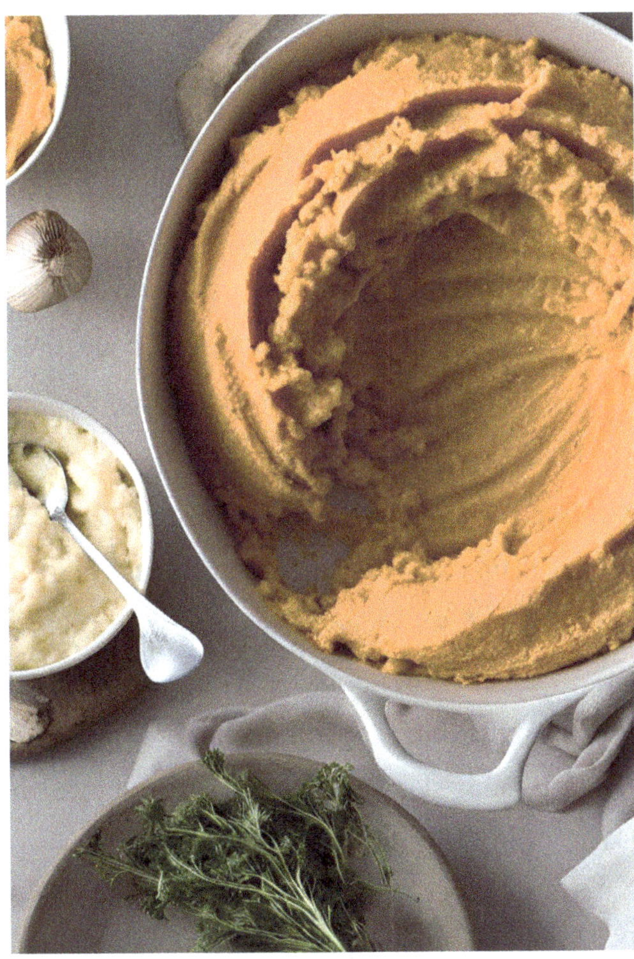

Time of Preparation: 10 minutes

Cooking Time: 20 minutes

Serving Units: 4

Ingredients:

- Two large piece of sweet potatoes, peeled and diced
- 3 cloves garlic, minced
- 2 tablespoons unsalted butter or olive oil
- 1/4 cup milk or non-dairy milk (such as almond milk or coconut milk)
- Salt and pepper to taste
- Fresh chives or parsley, chopped, for garnish (optional)

Procedures:

1. Place the cubed sweet potatoes in a large pot and cover them with water. Put the water over medium-high heat and bring it to a boil.
2. Reduce the heat to medium-low and simmer the sweet potatoes for 15-20 minutes, or until they are tender and easily pierced with a fork.
3. Drain the cooked sweet potatoes and transfer them to a large mixing bowl.
4. In the same pot used to cook the sweet potatoes, melt the butter or heat the olive oil over medium heat.
5. Add minced garlic to the pot and sauté for 1-2 minutes until fragrant and golden brown.
6. Remove the pot from heat and add the sautéed garlic, milk, salt, and pepper to the bowl with the cooked sweet potatoes.
7. Use a potato masher or fork to mash the sweet potatoes until smooth and creamy. Alternatively, you can use a

hand mixer or immersion blender for a smoother consistency.

8. Taste and adjust the seasoning as needed, adding more salt and pepper if desired.

9. Transfer the mashed sweet potatoes to a serving dish and garnish with chopped fresh chives or parsley if desired.

Nutritional Value (per serving):

- **Calories:** 150
- **Total Fat:** 5g
- **Saturated Fat:** 3g
- **Cholesterol:** 15mg
- **Sodium:** 80mg
- **Total Carbohydrates:** 25g
- **Dietary Fiber:** 4g
- **Sugars:** 7g
- **Protein:** 2g

Cooking Tips:

- Make sure to cut the sweet potatoes into evenly sized cubes to ensure they cook evenly and quickly.
- Be careful not to overcook the sweet potatoes, as they can become mushy and waterlogged. Test for doneness by piercing them with a fork; they should be tender but still hold their shape.
- Customize the mashed sweet potatoes by adding additional flavorings such as maple syrup, cinnamon, nutmeg, or a pinch of cayenne pepper for a hint of heat.
- For a dairy-free or vegan option, use olive oil or coconut oil instead of butter and non-dairy milk such as almond milk or coconut milk.
- If you prefer a smoother consistency, you can pass the mashed sweet potatoes through a fine-mesh sieve or potato ricer to remove any lumps.

Health Benefits:

1. **High in Vitamins and Minerals:** Sweet potatoes are rich in vitamins A, C, and B6, as well as potassium, manganese, and fiber, providing essential nutrients for overall health and well-being.

2. **Antioxidants:** Sweet potatoes are loaded with antioxidants such as beta-carotene, which help reduce inflammation, protect cells from damage caused by free radicals, and lower the risk of chronic diseases such as heart disease and cancer.

3. **Fiber-Rich:** Sweet potatoes are high in dietary fiber, which promotes digestive health, regulates bowel movements, and helps keep you feeling full and satisfied.

5

Snack Attack

AIP Trail Mix

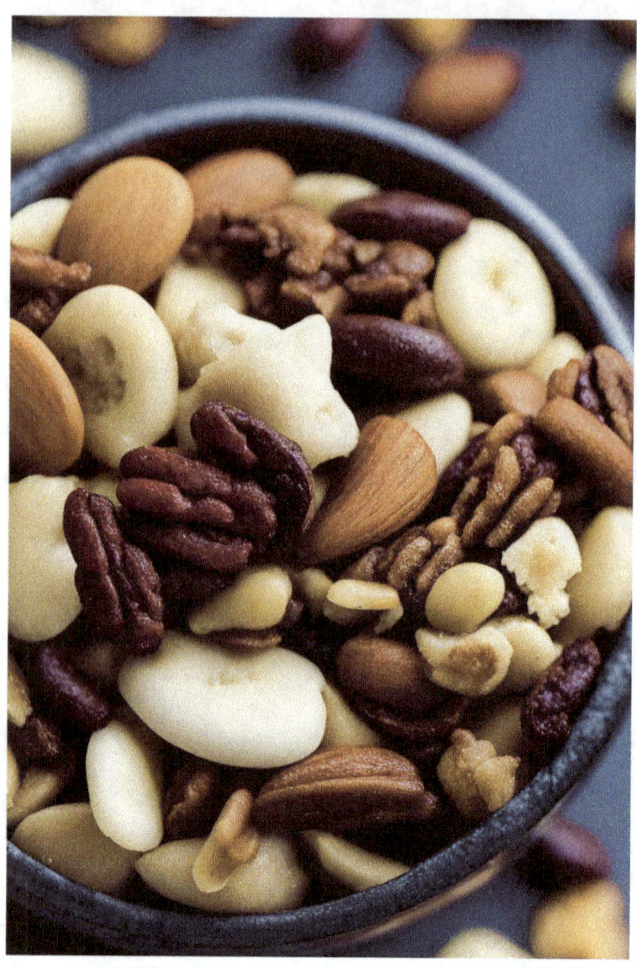

Time of Preparation: 10 minutes
Cooking Time: 0 minutes
Serving Units: Variable

Ingredients:

- 1 cup raw pumpkin seeds (pepitas)
- 1 cup raw sunflower seeds
- 1 cup unsweetened coconut flakes
- 1 cup dried cranberries (unsweetened and sulfur-free)
- 1/2 cup banana chips (unsweetened and sulfur-free)
- 1/2 cup dried apricots, chopped
- 1/2 cup dried figs, chopped
- 1/2 cup dried mango, chopped

Procedures:

1. In a large mixing bowl, combine all the ingredients: raw pumpkin seeds, raw sunflower seeds, unsweetened coconut flakes, dried cranberries, banana chips, chopped dried apricots, chopped dried figs, and chopped dried mango.
2. Ensure that all components are thoroughly combined and dispersed.
3. Transfer the trail mix to an airtight container or individual portion-sized bags for easy snacking.
4. Enjoy the AIP trail mix as a convenient and nutritious snack on the go, or sprinkle it over yogurt, smoothie bowls, or salads for added texture and flavor.

Nutritional Value (per serving, approximately 1/4 cup):

- **Calories:** 180
- **Total Fat:** 10g
- **Saturated Fat:** 4g
- **Cholesterol:** 0mg
- **Sodium:** 5mg

- **Total Carbohydrates:** 20g
- **Dietary Fiber:** 4g
- **Sugars:** 14g
- **Protein:** 4g

Cooking Tips:

- Customize the AIP trail mix by adding your favorite AIP-compliant ingredients such as dried blueberries, shredded coconut, tiger nuts, or Tigernut flour.
- Look for unsweetened and sulfur-free dried fruits to ensure they meet AIP guidelines and do not contain any added sugars, preservatives, or sulfites.
- Store the AIP trail mix in an airtight container in a cool, dry place to maintain freshness and prevent the seeds and fruits from becoming stale.
- Feel free to adjust the quantities of ingredients according to your preferences, adding more or less of each component to suit your taste.
- Check the labels of packaged ingredients to ensure they do not contain any non-compliant additives, such as added sugars, oils, or artificial flavors.

Health Benefits:

1. **Healthy Fats:** Pumpkin seeds, sunflower seeds, and coconut flakes are rich in healthy fats, including omega-3 and omega-6 fatty acids, which are important for brain health, heart health, and reducing inflammation in the body.
2. **Antioxidants:** Dried fruits are rich in antioxidants such as vitamin C and polyphenols, which help reduce inflammation, protect cells from damage caused by free radicals, and lower the risk of chronic diseases such as heart disease and cancer.
3. **Energy Boost:** The AIP trail mix provides a quick and convenient source of energy, making it an ideal snack for busy days, outdoor activities, or pre- and post-workout fuel.
4. **Blood Sugar Control:** The combination of healthy fats, fiber, and natural sugars in the AIP trail mix helps promote stable blood sugar levels, preventing spikes and crashes that can lead to cravings and energy fluctuations.

Baked Sweet Potato Chips

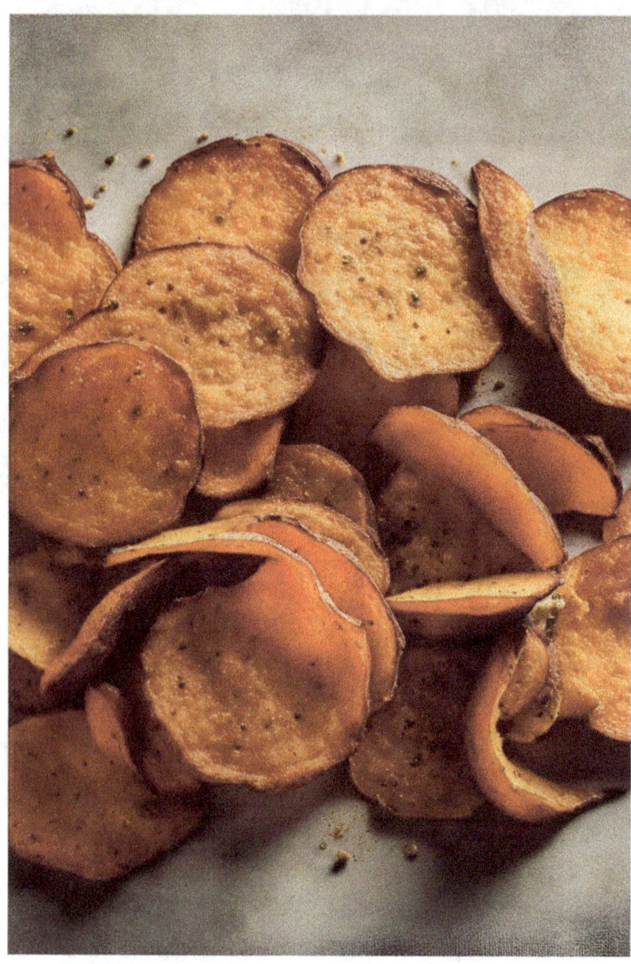

Time of Preparation: 15 minutes
Cooking Time: 20-25 minutes
Serving Units: 4

Ingredients:

- 2 large sweet potatoes, washed and thinly sliced (about 1/8 inch thick)
- 2 tablespoons olive oil
- 1 teaspoon paprika
- 1/2 teaspoon garlic powder
- 1/2 teaspoon onion powder
- Salt and pepper to taste
- Fresh parsley or rosemary, chopped, for garnish (optional)

Procedures:

1. Preheat the oven to 375°F (190°C). To make cleaning easier, line two baking pans with parchment paper.
2. In a large mixing bowl, toss the thinly sliced sweet potatoes with olive oil, paprika, garlic powder, onion powder, salt, and pepper until evenly coated.
3. Arrange the seasoned sweet potato slices in a single layer on the prepared baking sheets, making sure they do not overlap.
4. Bake in the preheated oven for 20-25 minutes, flipping the sweet potato chips halfway through the cooking time, until they are golden brown and crispy.
5. Remove the baking sheets from the oven and let the sweet potato chips cool for a few minutes before serving.
6. Garnish with chopped fresh parsley or rosemary if desired, and enjoy the baked sweet potato chips as a delicious and nutritious snack.

Nutritional Value (per serving):

- **Calories:** 120
- **Total Fat:** 7g
- **Saturated Fat:** 1g
- **Cholesterol:** 0mg
- **Sodium:** 150mg
- **Total Carbohydrates:** 14g
- **Dietary Fiber:** 2g
- **Sugars:** 5g
- **Protein:** 1g

Cooking Tips:

- Use a sharp knife or a mandoline slicer to thinly slice the sweet potatoes to ensure uniform thickness and even baking.
- Make sure to spread the sweet potato slices in a single layer on the baking sheets to allow for proper air circulation and crispy texture.
- Keep an eye on the sweet potato chips towards the end of the cooking time to prevent burning. They can go from golden brown to burnt quickly, so it's important to monitor them closely.
- Store any leftover baked sweet potato chips in an airtight container at room temperature for up to 2-3 days. They may lose some crispiness over time, but you can reheat them in the oven for a few minutes to revive their texture.

Health Benefits:

1. **Heart Health:** Sweet potatoes contain antioxidants such as beta-carotene and vitamin C, which help reduce inflammation, lower cholesterol levels, and support cardiovascular health.
2. **Healthy Fats:** Olive oil used for baking the sweet potato chips is rich in heart-healthy monounsaturated fats, which help lower bad cholesterol levels and reduce the risk of heart disease.
3. **Low Glycemic Index:** Sweet potatoes have a lower glycemic index compared to white potatoes, meaning they cause a slower and steadier rise in blood sugar levels, making them a ideal choice for people who are insulin resistant or have diabetes.
4. **Antioxidants:** The combination of sweet potatoes and olive oil provides a potent dose of antioxidants, which help reduce oxidative stress, protect cells from damage caused by free radicals, and reduce the chance of developing long-term illnesses including diabetes and cancer.

Guacamole with Veggie Sticks

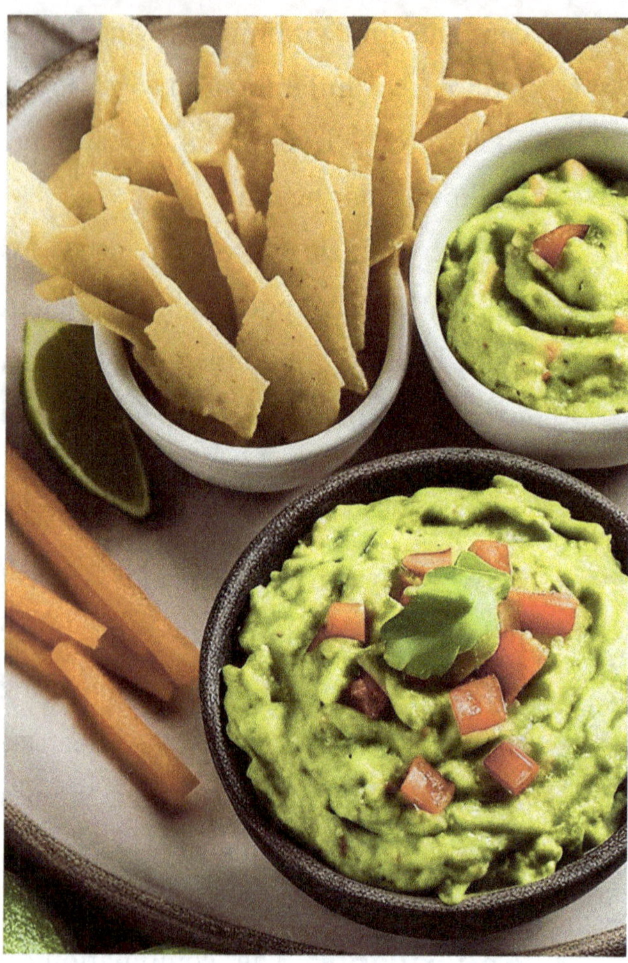

Time of Preparation: 15 minutes
Cooking Time: 0 minutes
Serving Units: 4

Ingredients:

- 2 ripe avocados
- 1 small tomato, diced
- 1/4 cup red onion, finely chopped
- 1 jalapeño pepper, seeded and minced (optional)
- 2 tablespoons fresh cilantro, chopped
- 1 lime, juiced
- Salt and pepper to taste
- Assorted vegetable sticks (carrots, celery, cucumber, bell peppers) for dipping

Procedures:

1. Cut the avocados in half, remove the pits, and scoop the flesh into a medium-sized mixing bowl.
2. Mash the avocados with a fork until smooth or leave them slightly chunky, depending on your preference.
3. Add diced tomato, finely chopped red onion, minced jalapeño pepper (if using), chopped cilantro, and lime juice to the mashed avocado.
4. Season the guacamole with salt and pepper to taste, and mix well to combine all the ingredients.
5. Taste the guacamole and adjust the seasoning or lime juice as needed.
6. Transfer the guacamole to a serving bowl and garnish with additional chopped cilantro or a slice of lime if desired.

7. Serve the guacamole with assorted vegetable sticks such as carrots, celery, cucumber, and bell peppers for dipping.

Nutritional Value (per serving, approximately 1/4 cup guacamole with veggie sticks):

- **Calories:** 150
- **Total Fat:** 12g
- **Saturated Fat:** 2g
- **Cholesterol:** 0mg
- **Sodium:** 10mg
- **Total Carbohydrates:** 10g
- **Dietary Fiber:** 6g
- **Sugars:** 2g
- **Protein:** 2g

Cooking Tips:

- Ripe avocados provide the greatest texture and flavor. They should yield slightly to gentle pressure when squeezed but should not be mushy.
- If you prefer a smoother guacamole, you can use a food processor or blender to blend the ingredients until smooth. Be careful not to over-blend, as you still want some texture in the guacamole.
- Customize the guacamole according to your taste preference by adding additional ingredients such as diced garlic, chopped green onions, or a pinch of cumin or chili powder.
- To prevent the guacamole from browning, store it in an airtight container with plastic wrap pressed directly onto the surface of the guacamole to minimize exposure to air. Alternatively, you can add a squeeze of additional lime juice on top before covering.
- For a spicier guacamole, leave the seeds in the jalapeño pepper or add a dash of hot sauce or cayenne pepper.
- Choose a variety of colorful vegetable sticks for dipping to add visual appeal and a range of nutrients. You can also serve the guacamole with whole-grain tortilla chips or pita bread for a heartier option.

Health Benefits:

1. **Heart-Healthy Fats:** Avocados are rich in monounsaturated fats, which help reduce bad cholesterol levels, lower the risk of heart disease, and support overall cardiovascular health.
2. **Dietary Fiber:** Avocados are high in dietary fiber, which promotes digestive health, regulates bowel movements, and helps keep you feeling full and satisfied.

3. **Vitamins and Minerals:** Avocados are packed with vitamins and minerals such as vitamin K, vitamin E, potassium, and folate, providing essential nutrients for overall health and well-being.

4. **Antioxidants:** Tomatoes, onions, and cilantro are rich in antioxidants such as vitamin C, lycopene, and quercetin, which help reduce inflammation, protect cells from damage caused by free radicals, and lower the risk of chronic diseases.

5. **Low in Sodium:** Guacamole is naturally low in sodium, making it a heart-healthy option for those watching their sodium intake or managing hypertension.

6. **Hydration:** Cucumbers and bell peppers are high in water content, helping to keep you hydrated and maintain optimal hydration levels throughout the day.

Cinnamon Apple Chips

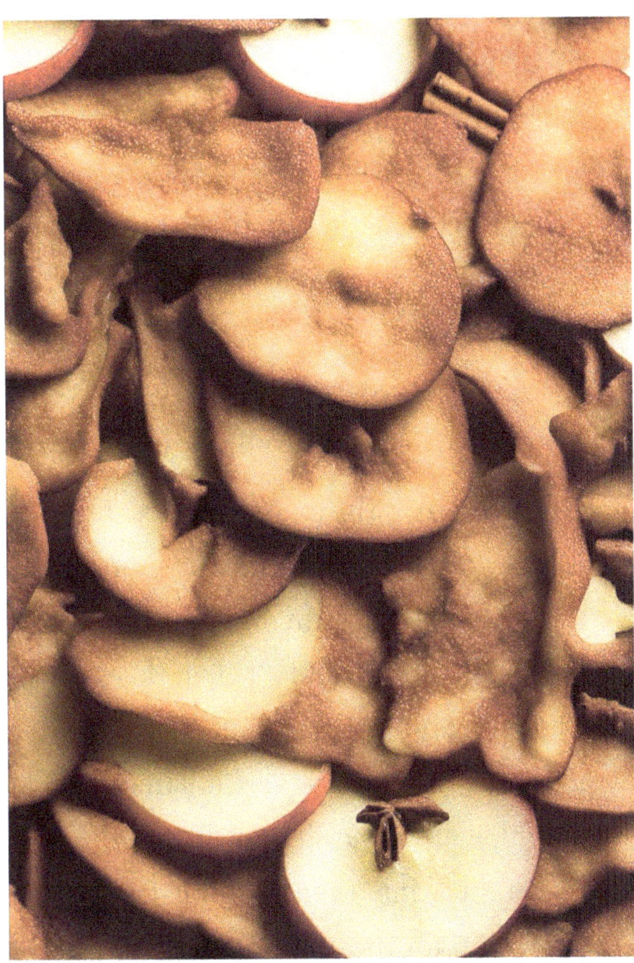

Time of Preparation: 15 minutes
Cooking Time: 2-3 hours
Serving Units: Variable

Ingredients:

- 2 large apples (such as Granny Smith or Fuji)
- 1 tablespoon ground cinnamon
- 1 tablespoon granulated sugar or coconut sugar (optional)

Procedures:

1. Preheat the oven to 200°F (95°C). To make cleaning easier, line two baking pans with parchment paper.
2. Wash and core the apples, then thinly slice them into rounds, about 1/8 inch thick, using a sharp knife or a mandoline slicer. Remove any seeds if necessary.
3. In a small bowl, mix together ground cinnamon and granulated sugar (if using).
4. Arrange the apple slices in a single layer on the prepared baking sheets, making sure they do not overlap.
5. Sprinkle the cinnamon sugar mixture evenly over the apple slices, coating them on both sides.
6. Bake the apple slices in the preheated oven for 2-3 hours, flipping them halfway through the cooking time, until they are dried and crispy.
7. Remove the baking sheets from the oven and let the cinnamon apple chips cool completely on the baking sheets before serving or storing.
8. Once cooled, transfer the cinnamon apple chips to an airtight container or resealable plastic bag for storage.

Nutritional Value (per serving, approximately 1/2 cup):

- **Calories:** 60
- **Total Fat:** 0g
- **Saturated Fat:** 0g
- **Cholesterol:** 0mg
- **Sodium:** 0mg
- **Total Carbohydrates: 16g**
- **Dietary Fiber:** 3g
- **Sugars:** 12g
- **Protein:** 0g

Cooking Tips:

- Choose firm and crisp apples such as Granny Smith or Fuji for the best results. These varieties hold their shape well during baking and provide a nice contrast to the sweet and spicy cinnamon flavor.
- Use a sharp knife or a mandoline slicer to thinly slice the apples into uniform rounds. This ensures even cooking and crispiness.
- To prevent the apple slices from browning, you can dip them in a mixture of lemon juice and water before sprinkling with cinnamon sugar.
- To avoid burning, keep a watch on the apple chips at the conclusion of the cooking process. They should be golden brown and crispy but not overly browned.
- Store the cinnamon apple chips in an airtight container at room temperature for up to 1 week. They may lose some crispiness over time, but you can reheat them in the oven for a few minutes to revive their texture.

Health Benefits:

1. **Rich in Fiber:** Apples are high in dietary fiber, which promotes digestive health, regulates bowel movements, and helps keep you feeling full and satisfied.
2. **Low in Calories:** Cinnamon apple chips are naturally low in calories and fat, making them a guilt-free snack option for those watching their calorie intake or trying to lose weight.
3. **Vitamins and Minerals:** Apples are packed with vitamins and minerals such as vitamin C, potassium, and antioxidants, providing essential nutrients for overall health and well-being.
4. **Antioxidants:** Cinnamon is rich in antioxidants such as polyphenols, which help reduce inflammation, lower blood sugar levels, and protect

against chronic diseases such as heart disease and cancer.

5. **Blood Sugar Control:** Cinnamon has been shown to improve insulin sensitivity and lower blood sugar levels, making it a beneficial spice for those with diabetes or insulin resistance.

6. **Portable and Convenient:** Cinnamon apple chips are a convenient and portable snack option for on-the-go, providing a healthy alternative to store-bought potato chips or candy.

AIP Guacamole with Plantain Chips

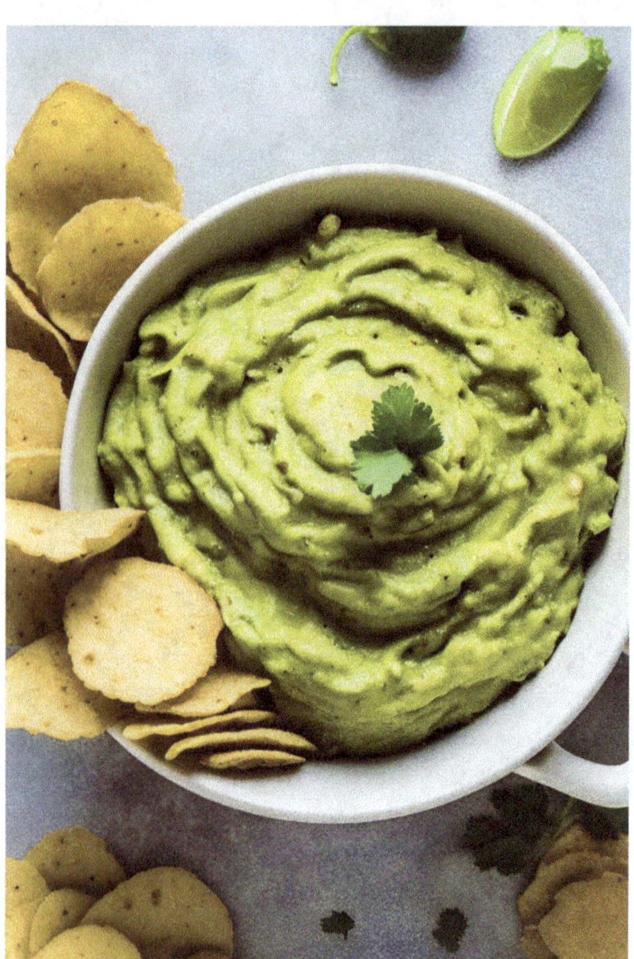

Time of Preparation: 20 minutes
Cooking Time: 20 minutes
Serving Units: 4

Ingredients: *For the Guacamole*:

- 2 ripe avocados
- 1 small tomato, diced
- 1/4 cup red onion, finely chopped
- 1/4 cup fresh cilantro, chopped
- 1 lime, juiced
- Salt to taste

For the Plantain Chips:

- 2 green plantains
- Two teaspoons of avocado or olive oil
- Sea salt to taste

Procedures: *For the Guacamole:*

1. Cut the avocados in half, remove the pits, and scoop the flesh into a mixing bowl.
2. Mash the avocados using a fork until desired consistency is reached.
3. Add diced tomato, finely chopped red onion, chopped cilantro, lime juice, and salt to the mashed avocados.
4. Mix all the ingredients until well combined. Adjust seasoning to taste.
5. Cover the guacamole and refrigerate until ready to serve.

For the Plantain Chips:

1. Preheat the oven to 375°F (190°C). Line a baking sheet with parchment paper.
2. Peel the plantains and thinly slice them using a mandoline slicer or a sharp knife.
3. In a mixing bowl, toss the plantain slices with olive oil until evenly coated.

4. Spread out the plantain slices on the baking sheet that has been prepared in a single layer.

5. Sprinkle sea salt over the plantain slices.

6. Bake in the preheated oven for 15-20 minutes, flipping halfway through, until the plantain chips are golden brown and crispy.

7. Remove from the oven and let cool before serving.

Nutritional Value (per serving):

- **Calories:** 200
- **Total Fat:** 15g
- **Saturated Fat:** 2g
- **Cholesterol:** 0mg
- **Sodium:** 150mg
- **Total Carbohydrates:** 20g
- **Dietary Fiber:** 5g
- **Sugars:** 8g
- **Protein:** 2g

Cooking Tips:

- Choose ripe avocados for the guacamole. They should yield to gentle pressure when squeezed but not be overly soft.
- Add diced red onion and chopped cilantro to the guacamole for added flavor and texture.

- Use fresh lime juice to enhance the flavor of the guacamole and prevent it from browning.
- Select green plantains for making plantain chips as they are firmer and less sweet than ripe plantains.
- Slice the plantains thinly and evenly to ensure even baking and crispiness.
- Toss the plantain slices in oil before baking to help them crisp up in the oven.
- Season the plantain chips with sea salt for a savory flavor.
- Keep an eye on the plantain chips while baking to prevent burning.

Health Benefits:

1. **Healthy Fats:** Rich in heart-healthy monounsaturated fats, avocados may help decrease harmful cholesterol levels.

2. **Vitamins and Minerals:** Avocados are a good source of vitamins C, E, K, and B vitamins, as well as potassium and folate.

3. **Antioxidants:** Plantains contain antioxidants such as vitamin C and flavonoids, which help protect cells from damage caused by free radicals.

4. **Fiber:** Both avocados and plantains are high in dietary fiber, which aids digestion and helps maintain a healthy weight.

5. **Gluten-Free and Paleo-Friendly:** This recipe is suitable for those following a gluten-free or paleo diet.

6. **Low Sodium:** Guacamole and plantain chips are naturally low in sodium, making them suitable for those watching their sodium intake.

6

Indulging treats

AIP Chocolate Avocado Mousse

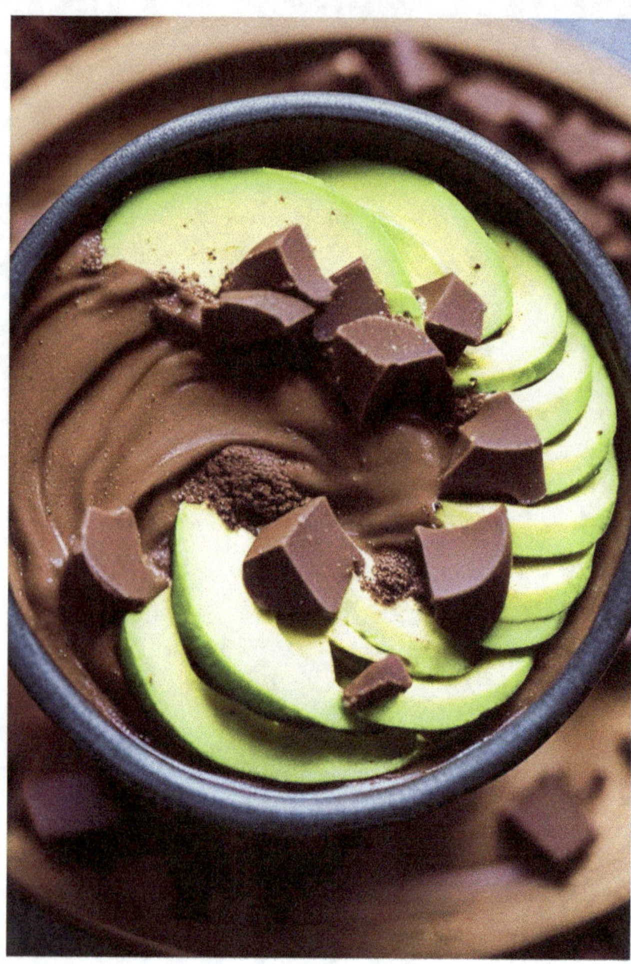

Time of Preparation: 10 minutes
Cooking Time: 0 minutes
Serving Units: 4

Ingredients:

- 2 ripe avocados
- 1/4 cup unsweetened cocoa powder
- 1/4 cup coconut milk (full fat)
- 1/4 cup maple syrup or honey (optional, adjust to taste)
- 1 teaspoon vanilla extract (optional)
- Pinch of salt

Procedures:

1. Cut the avocados in half, remove the pits, and scoop the flesh into a food processor or blender.
2. Add the unsweetened cocoa powder, coconut milk, maple syrup or honey (if using), vanilla extract (if using), and a pinch of salt to the avocados.
3. Blend the ingredients until smooth and creamy, scraping down the sides of the processor or blender as needed.
4. Taste the chocolate avocado mousse and adjust the sweetness or cocoa intensity by adding more maple syrup, cocoa powder, or vanilla extract if desired.
5. Once the desired consistency and flavor are achieved, transfer the chocolate avocado mousse to serving bowls or glasses.
6. Chill in the refrigerator for at least 30 minutes to allow the mousse to set and flavors to meld.
7. Serve the AIP chocolate avocado mousse chilled, garnished with fresh berries, shredded coconut, or a dollop of coconut whipped cream if desired.

Nutritional Value (per serving):

- **Calories:** 200
- **Total Fat:** 15g
- **Saturated Fat:** 3g
- **Cholesterol:** 0mg
- **Sodium:** 10mg
- **Total Carbohydrates:** 20g
- **Dietary Fiber:** 7g
- **Sugars:** 9g
- **Protein:** 3g

Cooking Tips:

- For the finest flavor and texture, choose ripe avocados. They should yield slightly to gentle pressure when squeezed but not be overly mushy.
- Use unsweetened cocoa powder to keep the chocolate avocado mousse AIP-compliant. Check the label to ensure there are no added sugars or dairy ingredients.
- For a richer and creamier texture, use full-fat coconut milk instead of light coconut milk.
- Adjust the sweetness of the mousse to your taste preferences by adding more or less maple syrup or honey. You can also use alternative sweeteners such as date syrup or coconut nectar.
- Add a splash of vanilla extract for extra flavor complexity, if desired. Make sure to use pure vanilla extract without any added sugar or alcohol.
- For a smooth and silky mousse, blend the ingredients thoroughly in a high-speed blender or food processor until no lumps remain.
- Chill the chocolate avocado mousse in the refrigerator for at least 30 minutes before serving to allow it to set and firm up.
- Serve the mousse topped with your favorite AIP-friendly toppings such as fresh berries, shredded coconut, chopped nuts, or a drizzle of melted dark chocolate.

Health Benefits:

1. **Heart-Healthy Fats:** Avocados are rich in monounsaturated fats, which help lower bad cholesterol levels and reduce the risk of heart disease.
2. **Antioxidants:** Cocoa powder is high in antioxidants such as flavonoids, which help reduce inflammation, improve blood flow, and protect cells from damage caused by free radicals.
3. **Dietary Fiber:** Avocados and cocoa powder are both high in dietary fiber, which promotes digestive health, regulates bowel movements, and helps keep you feeling full and satisfied.

4. **Blood Sugar Control:** Despite its sweet flavor, maple syrup or honey can be used sparingly to sweeten the mousse without causing significant spikes in blood sugar levels, making it suitable for those with diabetes or insulin resistance.

5. **Vitamins and Minerals:** Avocados are a good source of vitamins E, K, and B vitamins, as well as potassium and folate, providing essential nutrients for overall health and well-being.

6. **Satiety:** The combination of healthy fats and fiber in the chocolate avocado mousse helps promote satiety and prevent overeating, making it a satisfying and nourishing dessert option.

Coconut Milk Panna Cotta

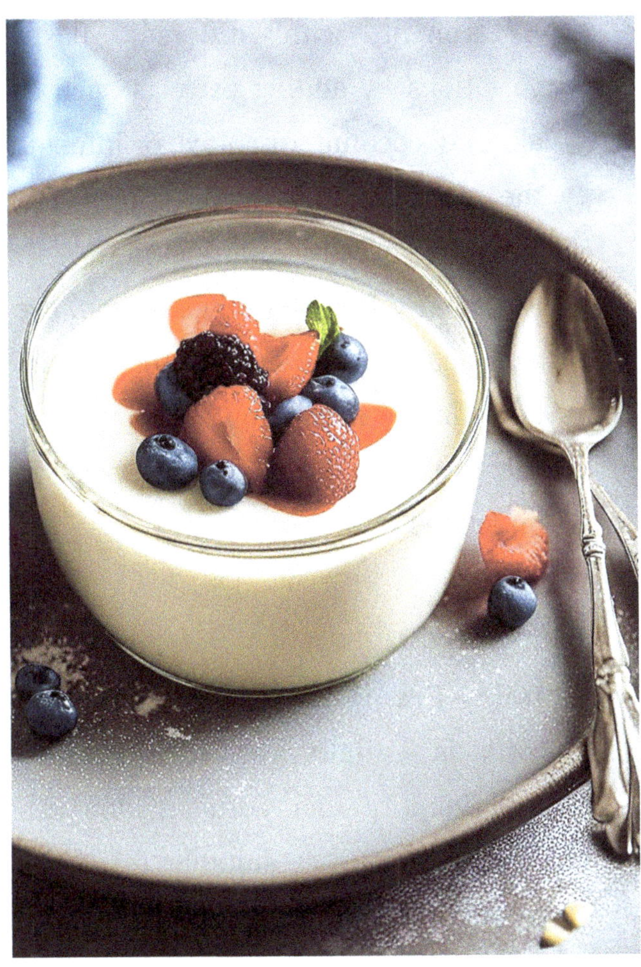

Time of Preparation: 10 minutes

Cooking Time: 5 minutes

Chilling Time: 4 hours

Serving Units: 4

Ingredients:

- Full-fat coconut milk, 1 (13.5 oz) can
- 2 tablespoons maple syrup or honey
- 1 teaspoon vanilla extract
- One package (2 1/4 tsp) of flavorless gelatin.
- 2 tablespoons cold water
- As a garnish, fresh berries or fruit compote are optional
- Shredded coconut or toasted nuts, for garnish (optional)

Procedures:

1. In a small bowl, sprinkle the unflavored gelatin over the cold water and let it sit for 5 minutes to bloom.
2. In a saucepan, heat the coconut milk over medium heat until warm but not boiling.
3. Stir in the maple syrup or honey and vanilla extract until well combined.
4. Add the bloomed gelatin to the warm coconut milk mixture and whisk until the gelatin is completely dissolved.
5. Take the pot off the burner and let the mixture to cool a little.
6. Pour the coconut milk panna cotta mixture into individual serving glasses or molds.
7. Cover the glasses or molds with plastic wrap and refrigerate for at least 4 hours, or until set.
8. Once set, remove the plastic wrap and garnish the coconut milk panna cotta with fresh berries, fruit compote,

shredded coconut, or toasted nuts if desired.

9. Serve chilled and enjoy!

Nutritional Value (per serving):

- **Calories:** 200
- **Total Fat:** 16g
- **Saturated Fat:** 14g
- **Cholesterol:** 0mg
- **Sodium:** 10mg
- **Total Carbohydrates:** 8g
- **Dietary Fiber:** 0g
- **Sugars:** 6g
- **Protein:** 2g

Cooking Tips:

- Use full-fat coconut milk to get a velvety, rich consistency. Shake the can well before opening to ensure the coconut cream and milk are well combined.
- Adjust the sweetness of the panna cotta to your taste preference by adding more or less maple syrup or honey.
- Make sure to dissolve the gelatin completely in the warm coconut milk mixture to avoid any lumps in the final dessert.
- To unmold the panna cotta easily, dip the bottom of the glasses or molds in warm water for a few seconds to loosen the edges before inverting onto serving plates.
- Experiment with different flavor variations by adding extracts such as almond, coconut, or coffee, or infusing the coconut milk with spices like cinnamon or cardamom.
- For a dairy-free and vegan option, use agar-agar powder instead of gelatin. For information on the proper substitution ratio, refer to the package directions.

Health Benefits:

1. **Dairy-Free:** Coconut milk panna cotta is a dairy-free alternative to traditional panna cotta made with cream, making it suitable for those with lactose intolerance or dairy allergies.
2. **Healthy Fats:** Coconut milk is rich in medium-chain triglycerides (MCTs), which are easily digested and may help boost metabolism and support weight loss.
3. **Low in Sugar:** Sweetened with maple syrup or honey, coconut milk panna cotta is lower in refined sugars compared to traditional desserts,

making it a healthier option for those watching their sugar intake.

4. **Gut Health:** Gelatin, derived from animal collagen, may support gut health by improving digestion, reducing inflammation, and strengthening the gut lining.

5. **Rich in Flavor:** Coconut milk adds a rich and creamy texture to the panna cotta while imparting a subtle coconut flavor, making it a delicious and indulgent dessert option.

6. **Versatile:** Coconut milk panna cotta can be customized with various toppings and flavorings to suit different tastes and preferences, making it a versatile dessert for any occasion.

Lemon Blueberry Muffins

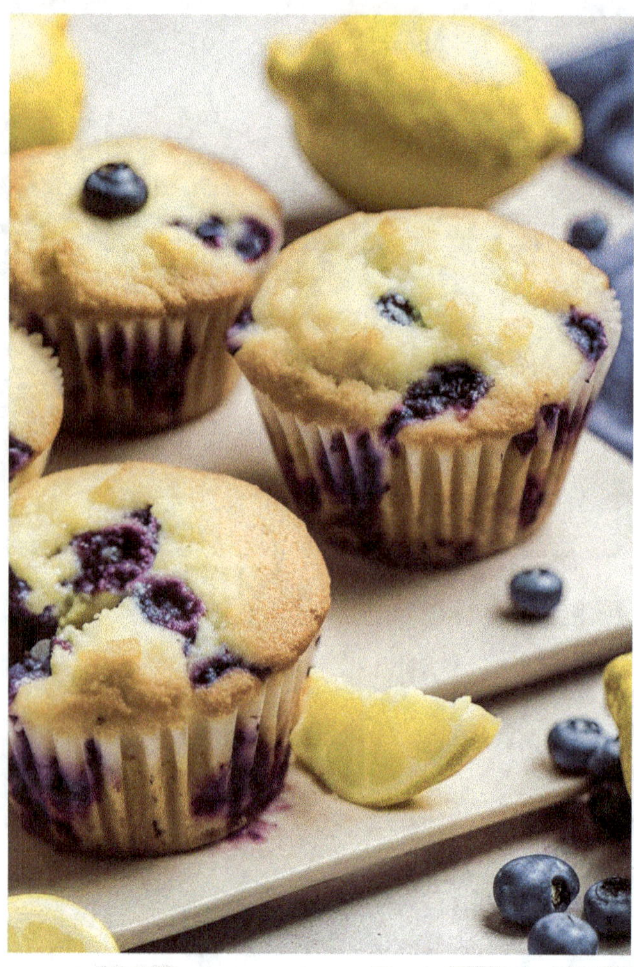

Time of Preparation: 15 minutes
Cooking Time: 20-25 minutes
Serving Units: 12

Ingredients:

- 2 cups all-purpose flour or almond flour (for gluten-free option)
- 1/2 cup granulated sugar or coconut sugar
- 2 teaspoons baking powder
- 1/2 teaspoon baking soda
- 1/4 teaspoon salt
- 1 cup plain Greek yogurt or coconut yogurt
- 1/4 cup unsalted butter or coconut oil, melted and cooled
- 2 large eggs
- 1 teaspoon vanilla extract
- Zest of 1 lemon
- 2 tablespoons fresh lemon juice
- 1 1/2 cups fresh or frozen blueberries

Procedures:

1. Preheat the oven to 375°F (190°C). Use cooking spray or paper liners to line a muffin tray.
2. Using a big mixing basin, thoroughly mix the flour, sugar, baking soda, baking powder, and salt.
3. In a separate bowl, whisk together the Greek yogurt, melted butter or coconut oil, eggs, vanilla extract, lemon zest, and lemon juice until smooth.
4. Add the liquid mixture to the dry mixture and whisk just until blended.
5. Gently fold in the blueberries until evenly distributed throughout the batter.

6. Divide the batter evenly among the prepared muffin cups, filling each cup about 3/4 full.

7. Optional: Sprinkle some extra sugar on top of each muffin for a crunchy topping.

8. Bake for 20 to 25 minutes in a preheated oven, or until a toothpick inserted into the middle comes out clean and the muffins are golden brown.

9. Remove the muffin tin from the oven and let the muffins cool in the tin for 5 minutes before transferring them to a wire rack to cool completely.

Nutritional Value (per muffin):

- **Calories:** 180
- **Total Fat:** 6g
- **Saturated Fat:** 3.5g
- **Cholesterol:** 45mg
- **Sodium:** 190mg
- **Total Carbohydrates:** 27g
- **Dietary Fiber:** 1g
- **Sugars:** 12g
- **Protein:** 5g

Cooking Tips:

- Almond flour may be substituted for all-purpose flour to make a gluten-free version. Adjust the baking time as almond flour tends to bake faster.

- Make sure the melted butter or coconut oil is cooled slightly before adding it to the wet ingredients to prevent cooking the eggs.

- Use fresh blueberries for the best flavor and texture, but frozen blueberries can be used as well. If using frozen blueberries, do not thaw them before adding to the batter to prevent excessive moisture.

- Do not overmix the batter to avoid tough and dense muffins. Mix until just combined to ensure tender and fluffy muffins.

- Lemon zest adds intense lemon flavor to the muffins, so do not skip it. Zest the lemon using a microplane or fine grater, taking care not to shred the bitter white pith.

- Adapt the sugar content to your personal taste preferences. You can use coconut sugar for a healthier option with a slightly caramelized flavor.

- To store leftover muffins, place them in an airtight container at room temperature for up to 2 days or in the refrigerator for up to 5 days. Moreover, they may be frozen for extended storage.

1. **Blueberries:** Rich in antioxidants, vitamins, and minerals, blueberries contribute to heart health, brain function, and may help reduce the risk of chronic diseases such as cancer.

2. **Greek Yogurt:** A good source of protein, calcium, and probiotics, Greek yogurt supports digestive health, strengthens bones, and promotes muscle growth and repair.

3. **Lemon:** High in vitamin C and antioxidants, lemons boost the immune system, aid digestion, and may help improve skin health and reduce inflammation.

4. **Eggs:** Packed with protein, vitamins, and minerals, eggs provide essential nutrients for muscle growth, brain function, and overall health.

5. **Almond Flour (if using):** Gluten-free and low in carbs, almond flour is high in healthy fats, fiber, and protein, making it suitable for those with gluten intolerance or following a low-carb diet.

Pumpkin Spice Energy Balls

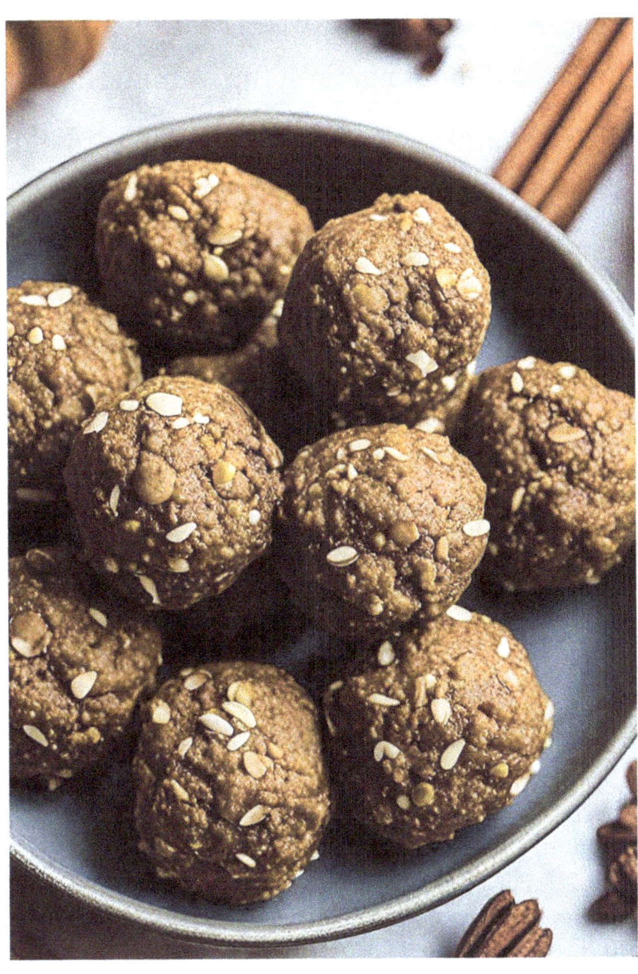

Time of Preparation: 15 minutes

Cooking Time: 0 minutes

Chilling Time: 30 minutes

Serving Units: Approximately 12 balls

Ingredients:

- 1 cup rolled oats
- 1/2 cup homemade or canned pureed pumpkin
- 1/4 cup almond butter or cashew butter
- 1/4 cup maple syrup or honey
- 1/4 cup unsweetened shredded coconut
- 1 teaspoon pumpkin pie spice
- 1/2 teaspoon vanilla extract
- Pinch of salt
- Optional add-ins: chopped nuts, raisins, dried cranberries, or chocolate chips

Procedures:

1. In a large mixing bowl, combine the rolled oats, pumpkin puree, almond butter or cashew butter, maple syrup or honey, shredded coconut, pumpkin pie spice, vanilla extract, and a pinch of salt.
2. Stir the ingredients until well combined. If the mixture seems too wet, add more rolled oats. If it's too dry, add a bit more pumpkin puree or nut butter.
3. Fold in any optional add-ins such as chopped nuts, raisins, dried cranberries, or chocolate chips for extra flavor and texture.
4. Once the mixture is well combined, use your hands to roll it into golf ball-sized energy balls. Wet your hands a

little with water if the mixture is too sticky to avoid sticking.

5. Place the energy balls on a baking sheet lined with parchment paper or a plate, and refrigerate for at least 30 minutes to firm up.

6. Once chilled, the pumpkin spice energy balls are ready to eat. Any leftovers can be kept in the fridge for up to a week if they are kept in an airtight container.

Nutritional Value (per ball):

- **Calories:** 100
- **Total Fat:** 5g
- **Saturated Fat:** 1g
- **Cholesterol:** 0mg
- **Sodium:** 20mg
- **Total Carbohydrates:** 12g
- **Dietary Fiber:** 2g
- **Sugars:** 5g
- **Protein:** 2g

Cooking Tips:

- Use rolled oats or old-fashioned oats for the best texture. Avoid using instant oats or steel-cut oats as they will not bind the energy balls together as well.

- Use pure pumpkin puree; avoid using pumpkin pie filling, which has additional spices and sugars.

- If you prefer a sweeter flavor, you can add more maple syrup or honey to the mixture. After tasting the combination, adjust the sweetness to your desired level.

- Customize the energy balls with your favorite add-ins such as chopped nuts, dried fruit, or chocolate chips. Use your imagination to try out various flavor and texture combinations.

- For a nut-free option, you can use sunflower seed butter or tahini instead of almond butter or cashew butter.

- If you don't have pumpkin pie spice on hand, you can make your own by combining ground cinnamon, nutmeg, ginger, and cloves.

- To make the rolling process easier, chill the mixture in the refrigerator for about 10-15 minutes before shaping into balls.

- Store the pumpkin spice energy balls in the refrigerator to keep them firm and prevent them from becoming too soft at room temperature.

1. **High in Fiber:** Rolled oats and pumpkin puree are both high in dietary fiber, which aids digestion, regulates blood sugar levels, and promotes satiety.

2. **Rich in Nutrients:** Pumpkin puree is packed with vitamins, minerals, and antioxidants, including vitamin A, vitamin C, potassium, and beta-carotene, which support immune function, eye health, and skin health.

3. **Healthy Fats:** Almond butter or cashew butter provide healthy fats, protein, and essential nutrients such as vitamin E and magnesium, which support heart health, brain function, and overall well-being.

4. **Natural Sweeteners:** Maple syrup or honey add sweetness to the energy balls without the need for refined sugars, providing a source of energy that is slow-releasing and less likely to cause blood sugar spikes.

5. **Convenient Snack:** Pumpkin spice energy balls are portable, convenient, and perfect for on-the-go snacking, providing a quick boost of energy and satisfaction whenever you need it.

6. **Versatile:** Energy balls are easily customizable with different flavors and add-ins, making them suitable for various dietary preferences and restrictions, including vegan, gluten-free, and dairy-free diets.

Berry Coconut Ice Cream

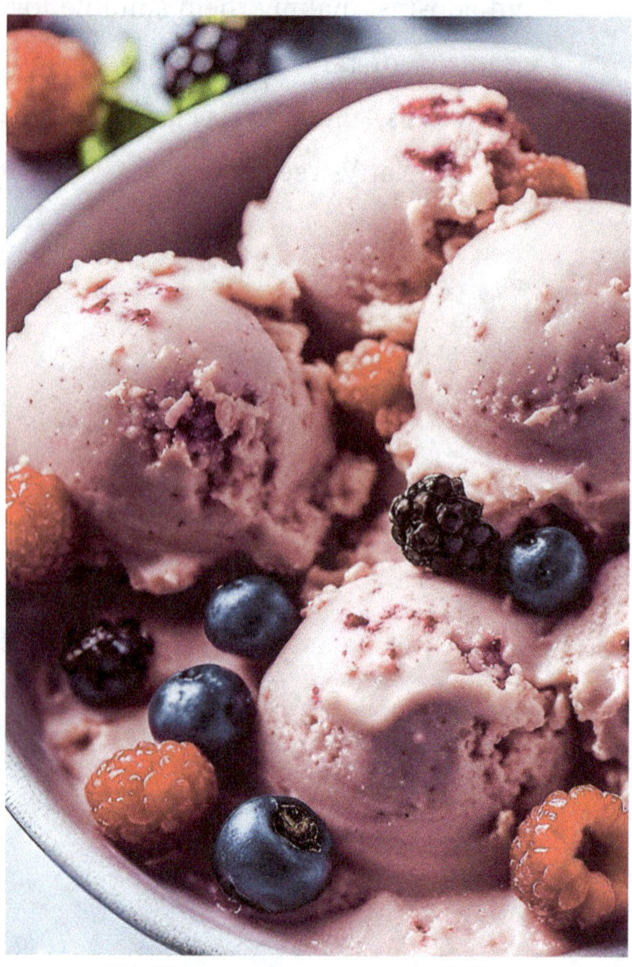

Time of Preparation: 10 minutes

Freezing Time: 4-6 hours

Serving Units: 4

Ingredients:

- 2 cups mixed berries (such as strawberries, blueberries, raspberries, and blackberries), fresh or frozen
- Full-fat coconut milk, 1 (13.5 oz) can
- 1/4 cup maple syrup or honey
- 1 teaspoon vanilla extract
- Pinch of salt

Procedures:

1. If using frozen berries, let them thaw slightly at room temperature for a few minutes.
2. In a blender or food processor, combine the mixed berries, coconut milk, maple syrup or honey, vanilla extract, and a pinch of salt.
3. Blend the mixture until smooth and creamy, scraping down the sides of the blender or food processor as needed.
4. Taste the mixture and adjust the sweetness or flavor as desired by adding more maple syrup, vanilla extract, or berries.
5. Once the mixture is smooth and well combined, transfer it to a shallow dish or loaf pan.
6. Cover the dish or pan with plastic wrap or a lid and place it in the freezer.
7. Freeze the berry coconut mixture for 4-6 hours, or until firm and scoopable.
8. When ready to serve, remove the dish or pan from the freezer and let the ice cream soften slightly at room temperature for a few minutes.

9. Scoop the berry coconut ice cream into bowls or cones and garnish with fresh berries or shredded coconut if desired.
10. Serve immediately and enjoy!

Nutritional Value (per serving):

- **Calories:** 200
- **Total Fat:** 15g
- **Saturated Fat:** 13g
- **Cholesterol:** 0mg
- **Sodium:** 10mg
- **Total Carbohydrates:** 18g
- **Dietary Fiber:** 3g
- **Sugars:** 12g
- **Protein:** 2g

Cooking Tips:

- Use a combination of your favorite berries for a variety of flavors and colors in the ice cream. Strawberries, blueberries, raspberries, and blackberries work well together.
- For a smoother texture, strain the berry mixture through a fine-mesh sieve to remove any seeds before freezing.
- Adjust the sweetness of the ice cream to your taste preference by adding more or less maple syrup or honey. Keep in mind that the sweetness may mellow slightly once frozen.
- If you prefer a creamier texture, you can add a few tablespoons of coconut cream or Greek yogurt to the mixture before freezing.
- To prevent ice crystals from forming, give the ice cream mixture a stir every hour or so during the freezing process.
- For a faster freezing time, spread the mixture into a thin layer on a baking sheet lined with parchment paper before freezing. Once frozen, break the mixture into chunks and blend again until smooth before serving.
- Store any leftover ice cream in an airtight container in the freezer for up to one week. Before scooping, let it soften for a few minutes at room temperature.

Health Benefits:

1. **Antioxidants:** Berries are rich in antioxidants such as anthocyanins and vitamin C, which help protect cells from damage caused by free radicals and may reduce the risk of chronic diseases.
2. **Healthy Fats:** Coconut milk provides healthy fats called medium-chain triglycerides (MCTs), which are easily

digested and may support heart health, brain function, and weight management.

3. **Natural Sweeteners:** Maple syrup or honey adds sweetness to the ice cream without the need for refined sugars, providing a source of energy that is slow-releasing and less likely to cause blood sugar spikes.

4. **Dietary Fiber:** Berries and coconut milk are both high in dietary fiber, which supports digestive health, regulates blood sugar levels, and promotes satiety.

5. **Vitamins and Minerals:** Berries are a good source of vitamins A, C, and K, as well as folate and potassium, while coconut milk provides essential nutrients such as manganese, copper, and selenium.

6. **Dairy-Free:** This ice cream is dairy-free, making it suitable for individuals with lactose intolerance or dairy allergies, as well as those following a vegan or plant-based diet.

Conclusion

As you reach the end of this journey through the autoimmune protocol (AIP) lifestyle, take a moment to reflect on how far you've come and the progress you've made in managing your autoimmune condition. From the moment you embarked on this path, you committed yourself to prioritizing your health and well-being, and that dedication has brought you to where you are today.

Throughout this book, you've learned about the principles of the AIP, the importance of nutrient-dense foods, the role of mindfulness and stress reduction, and the benefits of physical activity in managing autoimmune symptoms. Armed with this knowledge, you've embraced a new way of eating, living, and caring for yourself—one that empowers you to take control of your health and live life to the fullest.

Maintaining Long-Term Health and Wellness

As you move forward on your AIP journey, remember that this is not just a short-term diet but a long-term commitment to your health and well-being. While it may have started as a means to manage autoimmune symptoms, the AIP has likely become much more than that—it's a way of life, a philosophy, and a mindset that shapes your choices and priorities each day.

To maintain long-term health and wellness, continue to nourish your body with nutrient-dense foods, prioritize self-care and stress management, stay active and engaged in physical activity, and cultivate a supportive community of friends, family, and healthcare professionals who understand and support your journey.

Embracing a New Lifestyle

Embracing the AIP lifestyle means embracing a new way of thinking, eating, and living—one that puts your health and well-being first, above all else. It means making conscious choices that support your body's needs and honor your unique journey. It means finding joy and satisfaction in nourishing foods, mindful practices, and meaningful connections with others.

As you navigate the ups and downs of life with autoimmune disease, remember that you are not alone. There is a vast community of individuals who understand what you're going through and are here to support and encourage you every step of the way. Together, we can inspire each other, share our experiences, and empower one another to live our best lives despite the challenges we face.

Words of Encouragement and Inspiration

In closing, I want to offer you some words of encouragement and inspiration as you continue on your AIP journey:

You are stronger than you think, and more resilient than you realize. Every day, you have the opportunity to make choices that support your health and well-being, and every step you take brings you closer to your goals.

Be patient with yourself, and trust in the process. Healing takes time, and there will be ups and downs along the way. But with determination, perseverance, and a positive mindset, you can overcome any obstacle and achieve the vibrant health and vitality you deserve.

Remember to celebrate your successes, no matter how small, and to be kind to yourself when things don't go as planned. Each day is a new opportunity to start fresh, to learn and grow, and to embrace the beauty and possibility of life.

You are worthy of love, of joy, and of all the blessings life has to offer. So, keep moving forward with courage and conviction, knowing that you are on the path to greater health, happiness, and fulfillment than you ever thought possible.

With deepest gratitude and admiration for your strength and resilience,

Grace Mitchell

28-Days Meal Plan

Week 1

Day 1:

- **Breakfast:** Coconut Flour Pancakes
- **Lunch:** Avocado Chicken Salad
- **Dinner:** Herb-Crusted Salmon
- **Snack:** AIP Trail Mix

Day 2:

- **Breakfast:** Berry Smoothie Bowl
- **Lunch:** Roasted Beet and Arugula Salad
- **Dinner:** Garlic and Herb Roasted Vegetables
- **Snack:** Baked Sweet Potato Chips

Day 3:

- **Breakfast:** Turmeric Ginger Smoothie
- **Lunch:** Spinach and Strawberry Salad
- **Dinner:** Lemon Garlic Chicken Thighs
- **Snack:** Guacamole with Veggie Sticks

Day 4:

- **Breakfast:** AIP Breakfast Bowl
- **Lunch:** Kale and Chicken Caesar Salad with Avocado Dressing
- **Dinner:** Turkey and Sweet Potato Skillet
- **Snack:** Cinnamon Apple Chips

Day 5:

- **Breakfast:** Sweet Potato Hash
- **Lunch:** Roasted Butternut Squash Soup
- **Dinner:** Cauliflower Rice Stir-Fry
- **Snack:** AIP Guacamole with Plantain Chips

Day 6:

- **Breakfast:** Healing Bone Broth Soup
- **Lunch:** AIP Vegetable Stew
- **Dinner:** Herb-Crusted Salmon
- **Snack:** AIP Chocolate Avocado Mousse

Day 7:

- **Breakfast:** Turmeric Chicken Soup
- **Lunch:** Avocado Chicken Salad
- **Dinner:** Garlic Mashed Sweet Potatoes
- **Snack:** Berry Coconut Ice Cream

Week 2

Day 8:

- **Breakfast:** Coconut Flour Pancakes
- **Lunch:** Roasted Beet and Arugula Salad
- **Dinner:** Lemon Garlic Chicken Thighs
- **Snack:** Baked Sweet Potato Chips

Day 9:

- **Breakfast:** Berry Smoothie Bowl
- **Lunch:** Spinach and Strawberry Salad
- **Dinner:** Turkey and Sweet Potato Skillet
- **Snack:** Guacamole with Veggie Sticks

Day 10:

- **Breakfast:** Turmeric Ginger Smoothie
- **Lunch:** Kale and Chicken Caesar Salad with Avocado Dressing
- **Dinner:** Garlic and Herb Roasted Vegetables
- **Snack:** Cinnamon Apple Chips

Day 11:

- **Breakfast:** AIP Breakfast Bowl
- **Lunch:** Roasted Butternut Squash Soup
- **Dinner:** Herb-Crusted Salmon
- **Snack:** AIP Guacamole with Plantain Chips

Day 12:
• **Breakfast:** Sweet Potato Hash
• **Lunch:** AIP Vegetable Stew
• **Dinner:** Cauliflower Rice Stir-Fry
• **Snack:** AIP Chocolate Avocado Mousse
Day 13:
• **Breakfast:** Healing Bone Broth Soup
• **Lunch:** Avocado Chicken Salad
• **Dinner:** Lemon Garlic Chicken Thighs
• **Snack:** Berry Coconut Ice Cream
Day 14:
• **Breakfast:** Turmeric Chicken Soup
• **Lunch:** Roasted Beet and Arugula Salad
• **Dinner:** Turkey and Sweet Potato Skillet
• **Snack:** AIP Trail Mix

Week 3

Day 15:
• **Breakfast:** Coconut Flour Pancakes
• **Lunch:** Spinach and Strawberry Salad
• **Dinner:** Garlic and Herb Roasted Vegetables
• **Snack:** Baked Sweet Potato Chips
Day 16:
• **Breakfast:** Berry Smoothie Bowl
• **Lunch:** Kale and Chicken Caesar Salad with Avocado Dressing
• **Dinner:** Herb-Crusted Salmon
• **Snack:** Guacamole with Veggie Sticks
Day 17:
• **Breakfast:** Turmeric Ginger Smoothie
• **Lunch:** Roasted Butternut Squash Soup
• **Dinner:** Lemon Garlic Chicken Thighs

• **Snack:** Cinnamon Apple Chips

Day 18:

- **Breakfast:** AIP Breakfast Bowl
- **Lunch:** AIP Vegetable Stew
- **Dinner:** Turkey and Sweet Potato Skillet
- **Snack:** AIP Guacamole with Plantain Chips

Day 19:

- **Breakfast:** Sweet Potato Hash
- **Lunch:** Avocado Chicken Salad
- **Dinner:** Cauliflower Rice Stir-Fry
- **Snack:** AIP Chocolate Avocado Mousse

Day 20:

- **Breakfast:** Healing Bone Broth Soup
- **Lunch:** Roasted Beet and Arugula Salad
- **Dinner:** Garlic Mashed Sweet Potatoes
- **Snack:** Berry Coconut Ice Cream

Day 21:

- **Breakfast:** Turmeric Chicken Soup
- **Lunch:** Spinach and Strawberry Salad
- **Dinner:** Herb-Crusted Salmon
- **Snack:** AIP Trail Mix

Week 4

Day 22:

- **Breakfast:** Coconut Flour Pancakes
- **Lunch:** Kale and Chicken Caesar Salad with Avocado Dressing
- **Dinner:** Lemon Garlic Chicken Thighs
- **Snack:** Baked Sweet Potato Chips

Day 23:

- **Breakfast:** Berry Smoothie Bowl
- **Lunch:** Roasted Butternut Squash Soup

• **Dinner:** Turkey and Sweet Potato Skillet
• **Snack:** Guacamole with Veggie Sticks
Day 24:
• **Breakfast:** Turmeric Ginger Smoothie
• **Lunch:** AIP Vegetable Stew
• **Dinner:** Garlic and Herb Roasted Vegetables
• **Snack:** Cinnamon Apple Chips
Day 25:
• **Breakfast:** AIP Breakfast Bowl
• **Lunch:** Avocado Chicken Salad
• **Dinner:** Herb-Crusted Salmon
• **Snack:** AIP Guacamole with Plantain Chips
Day 26:
• **Breakfast:** Sweet Potato Hash
• **Lunch:** Roasted Beet and Arugula Salad
• **Dinner:** Cauliflower Rice Stir-Fry
• **Snack:** AIP Chocolate Avocado Mousse
Day 27:
• **Breakfast:** Healing Bone Broth Soup
• **Lunch:** Spinach and Strawberry Salad
• **Dinner:** Lemon Garlic Chicken Thighs
• **Snack:** Berry Coconut Ice Cream
Day 28:
• **Breakfast:** Turmeric Chicken Soup
• **Lunch:** Kale and Chicken Caesar Salad with Avocado Dressing
• **Dinner:** Turkey and Sweet Potato Skillet
• **Snack:** AIP Trail Mix

This 28-day meal plan incorporates a variety of recipes to ensure you enjoy different flavors and nutrients each day. Each meal is designed to be AIP compliant, balancing protein, healthy fats, and plenty of fruits and vegetables.